GIANT CELLS AND GIANT CELL LESIONS OF ORAL CAVITY

By

Dr Shikha Saxena
Professor, Department of Oral Pathology and Microbiology, RUHS College of Dental Sciences , Jaipur

Dr Priyanka Singh
Additional professor, Oral Pathology King George's Medical University, Shahmina Road, Chowk, Lucknow

EDSOL

Published by **EDSOL INFORMATICS**
Plot No 9, Add India Center Building,
7th floor, Supreme work, Sector 125,
Noida, Uttar Pradesh 201303

ISBN: 978-81-984958-6-0
First Edition: 202

GIANT CELLS AND GIANT CELL LESIONS OF ORAL CAVITY

Dr Shikha Saxena; Dr Priyanka Singh

For more information regarding **EDSOL INFORMATICS** and its products, please visit the publisher's website
www.edsolinformatics.com

Forward

With more than 10 years of experience in treating oral and maxillofacial lesions, the giant cells lesions of oral cavity are frequently encountered. The proper diagnosis of lesion is very important in determining the prognosis of the lesion.

The author is having an extensive experience in the subject of Oral Pathology and has beautifully described the multinucleate giant cells with detailed description of types, classification and mechanism of formation of giant cells. The book also focuses on giant cell lesions; their clinical features, radiographic features and histopathologic features and treatment modalities.

Dr. Sonal Priya Bhansali,

Professor,

Department of Oral Surgery,

RUHS College of Dental Sciences, Jaipur.

Preface

Multinucleated giant cells are morphologically characterized by the presence of multiple nuclei dispersed in cytoplasm. Foreign body giant cells, Langhan's giant cells, Touton giant cells, tumour giant cells, are various types of giant cells apart from the miscellaneous types of giant cells such as Aschoff cells of rheumatic nodule and Reed Sternberg cells of Hodgkin's lymphoma. Multinucleated cells are commonly encountered in oral and maxillofacial lesions..

A number of cystic, metabolic, osteodystrophic, microbial, tumour and tumour like lesions of the oral cavity present with characteristic giant cell lesions; which makes their diagnosis and study simpler. We have attempted to classify and review the common giant cells and giant cell lesions of the oral cavity, giving a brief account of their clinical, histological and diagnostic features, along with their recent treatment modalities.

ACKNOWLEDGEMENT

My heartfelt thanks to my teacher, parents, husband and my dearest daughters Mishi and Shivi without whom this book could not have been possible.

Table of Contents

UNIT 1
INTRODUCTION

Inflammation consists of vascular response, migration and activation of leukocytes and systemic reactions and is a response to various injurious agents such as microorganisms and necrotic cells. Inflammation can be of two types: acute and chronic. Acute inflammation is an immediate adaptive response of limited duration. It is mediated by activation of range of vasoactive and chemtactic pathways which result in local vasodilatation, with increased blood flow to affected area, resulting in increased vascular permeability and exudation of the fluid and plasma proteins (edema) and the emigration of leukocytes, predominantly neutrophils.[1]

Chronic inflammation is a biologically distinct pattern of response characterized by simultaneous inflammation and repair. It is of longer duration and is associated histologically with the presence of lymphocytes and macrophages, the proliferation of blood vessels, fibrosis and tissue necrosis, and is regulated by complex interaction between cytokines and growth factors.[1]

It is hypothesized, that when the macrophages (also called scavenger cell) are not able to deal with the noxious stimuli to be removed, they fuse together and form multinucleated giant cells. Multinucleated giant cells are found in many chronic infective granulomas. Giant cells may be found at the site of old haemorrhages and are also associated with attempted removal of cholesterol crystals. The lesion of traumatic fat necrosis often shows numerous giant cells.[2]

Giant cell lesions of oral tissues are a diverse group of lesions which are little understood and in recent years have been an object of clinical, histological and especially ultra structural investigations. The giant cell lesions owe their name to the presence of multinucleated giant cells seen on histopathological examination.

MULTINUCLEATED GIANT CELLS

Rokitansky and Langhans in 1868 first reported multinucleate giant cells in tuberculous granulomas. These cells are also known as polykaryocytes or syncytium. These cells have cytoplasm with multiple nuclei and are not divided into cells.[3]

Borrel (1893) was the first to suggest that multinucleated giant cells are fused masses of mononuclear leucocytes. Observation of tissues under the microscope allows the generalization that cells normally contain a single nucleus. This broad generalization is broken in a relatively small number of specific circumstances. Some tissues regularly contain cells in which several nuclei share the same cytoplasm: skeletal muscle, placenta and bone. The occurrence of polykaryons elsewhere is always abnormal. By far the most commonly observed is the inflammatory giant cell (macrophage polykaryon), which appears regularly in response to a wide variety of stimuli.[4]

These giant cells are now recognized as a common feature of granulomas induced both by immunological and non-immunological stimuli. Thus, they are found in granulomas associated with the immune response to tuberculosis, leprosy, syphilis, and various fungal and parasitic infections as well as in granulomas associated with nonimmune responses to toxic agents such as silica, beryllium, and asbestos, nontoxic agents such as carbon particles, plastic beads, and iron particles.[3]

Nevertheless, the origin and the mechanism of the formation of multinucleated giant cells is still not clear. It is possible, as different immune and non- immunological stimuli produce granulomas, that these multinucleate giant cells are formed by several different mechanisms. Thus, they may arise from the fusion of nonreplicating monocytes or from the mitotic and amitotic division of monocyte nuclei in the absence of cellular division. Several observations suggest that cellular immune mechanisms play a direct role. The giant cells have been found in granulomas of the skin produced by delayed hypersensitivity reactions in humans and in experimental animals.[5]

There is controversy regarding the formation of the multinucleated giant cells in the giant cell granuloma. Adkins suggested that the giant cells are formed by the fusion of the stromal cells, while others support the fact that they originate from endothelial cells of capillaries, fibroblasts or myofibroblasts.[5]

UNIT 2
GIANT CELL

Classification of Multinucleated Giant Cells- by **T.J. Chambers** (1978)[4]

A) Inflammatory Giant cell

B) Osteoclasts

C) Tumor Associated Multinucleated Giant Cell

D) Miscellaneous Multinucleated Giant Cell

Classification of Multinucleated Giant Cells- According to their occurrence in the body:

1. **Physiologic state:**
    - a) Osteoclasts
2. **Pathological state:**
    - A) Damaged striated muscle fibres:
        - i) Regenerating sarcolemmal cells in damaged voluntary muscle
        - ii) Aschoff giant cells in heart muscle (fused myocardial macrophages)
    - B) Fused fibroblast: (Giant Cell Fibroma)
    - C) Fused Macrophages:
        - i)Due to reaction to foreign bodies (exogenous or endogenous materials) E.g.Foreign body giant cells with scattered nuclei.
        - ii)Due to reaction to organisms as in tuberculosis and fungal infections

          E.g. - Langhan's giant cell in tuberculosis
        - iii)Touton giant cells of Xanthoma
    - D) Fused cells due to viral infections:
        - i) Epithelial giant cells as in HSV infections
        - ii) Connective tissue cells as in measles (Warthin Finkeldey Cells)
    - E) Tumor giant cells:
        - i) Reed Sternberg cells in Hodgkin's lymphoma

ii) Giant cells in Central giant cell granuloma, Poorly differentiated astrocytoma

iii) Giant cells in other tumors e.g. Carcinoma, Malignant fibrous histocytoma

Inflammatory Giant Cell

These multinucleate giant cells are commonly seen in pathologic material. They regularly appear as part of the response to the presence in tissues of a variety of foreign or insoluble substances. Because of this association and because they often contain ingested material they are generally assumed to represent a specialisation for improved phagocytosis. They have, however, been shown to have a poor phagocytic performance (Papadimitriou, Robertson and Walters, 1975; Chambers 1977).[4]

Some conditions associated with macrophage giant cell formation-[4]

a) Deposition or implantation of poorly soluble sterile materials in the tissues- Lipids, oils, cholesterol, glass, cellophane, agar, talc, sutures, uric acid, keratin, beryllium, silica, barium.

b) Infective granulomas- Tuberculosis, leprosy, syphilis, fungal diseases, lymphogranuloma venereum, cat scratch.

c) Granulomatous diseases of unknown etiology – Sarcoidosis, giant cell arteritis, wegner's granulomatosis, crohn's disease, rheumatic fever, rheumatoid nodules.

Morphological variants of inflammatory giant cells-[4]

i. The polykaryocyte described by Langhans (1868), showed a granular mass in the centre with circular peripheral arrangement.

ii. Mariano and Spector (1974) showed the foreign body giant cells, the nuclei of which are scattered in an irregular fashion throughout the cell.

iii. Haythorn (1929) described the intermediate type; these are the cells possessing a nuclear arrangement between these two types.

Roizman (1962) suggested that the morphological variants presumably represent different phases in the life of the same cell.[6]

Lambert (1912) in a series of in-vitro experiments with chicken spleen cells, observed the formation of multinucleate giant cells from wandering mononuclear phagocytes. Some years later the Lewises (1925, 1927) reported the transformation of large mononuclear leucocytes from the blood of elasmobranchs, teleosts, amphibian, reptiles, birds and mammals, into multinucleate giant cells in hanging drop cultures. Gillman and Wright (1966) presented data which strongly suggested that the multinucleate giant cells in inflammatory granulomas formed from circulating mononuclears which they had labelled with tritriated thymidine. It can thus be concluded that the mononuclear phagocyte is the precursor of inflammatory giant cells.[4]

At one time, it was customary to differentiate between polykaryocytes in lesions caused by sterile foreign bodies and the polykaryocytes named after Langhans which are found chiefly in infective granulomas. Both Langhans and foreign body multinucleate giant cells, however, may be found in both infective and sterile granulomas.[4]

The foreign body giant cell:

Giant cell formation can be seen around a foreign body such as fragment of bone. Such cells are called as foreign body giant cell (FBGC).[2] The most common foreign body granuloma is the suture granuloma, in which the macrophages and foreign body giant cells are present at the surface of the suture and this layer of cells is encapsulated in fibroconnective tissue, i.e., the fibrous capsule.[7]

The foreign body giant cell contain numerous nuclei (up to 100) which are uniform in size and shape and resemble nuclei of macrophages, these nuclei are scattered throughout the cytoplasm. They are formed as a reaction to exogenous insoluble material (talc, silica, ligature etc.) or to insoluble materials formed in the body (keratin, sodium urate crystals, cholesterol and fat), or reaction to certain organisms (tuberculosis, fungal infections, syphillis).[2]

The foreign body giant cell is a very large cell formed by the fusion of multiple macrophages, typically epitheloid cells. The stimulus for fusion is a foreign particle that is too large for phagocytosis by one macrophage or has mechanisms to negate phagocytosis and killing mechanisms. The giant cell exhibits multiple nuclei, often arranged in the periphery of the cell, and can measure up to 60 micrometres in diameter.[8]

The foreign body giant cells are found at the core of granulomas produced by granulomatous inflammation. In foreign body granulomas there seems to be a strong stimulus for fusion, since the fusion index is high and the foreign body type of giant cells predominates.[8]

Human Interleukin-4 induces the formation of FBGCs from human monocyte-derived macrophages, an effect that is optimized with either granulocyte-macrophage colony-stimulating factor (GM CSF) or Interleukin-3, dependent on the concentration of Interleukin-4, and specifically prevented by Anti Interleukin-4.[7]

Langhans type of giant cells:

Langhans giant cells are named for **Theodor Langhans** (1839-1915), a German pathologist, who first described these cells in 1868.[2]

The histiocytes belong to the reticuloendothelial system, although to the wandering members of that group. These large polyhedral cells, being designed for phagocytosis have abundant cytoplasm. Epitheloid cells are merely histiocytes with abundant pale cytoplasm like that of epithelium. The lipid content may be high accounting for the abundance and pallor of the cytoplasm. The epitheloid cells have a tendency to fuse forming large multinucleated giant cells of the foreign body or Langhans type.[2]

Langhans giant cells are characterized by the presence of small numbers of nuclei (<20) arranged peripherally within the giant cell, are commonly found in immune granulomas in granulomatous inflammations. Immune granulomas with the presence of Langhans giant cells are commonly formed in the presence of indigestible particles of organisms, e.g., the tubercle bacillus, and T cell-mediated immunity to the inciting agent. *In vivo* and *in vitro* experiments have suggested a role for interferon-γ in immune granuloma formation, although conflicting results have been reported. Among cytokines inducing monocyte-macrophage fusion, interferon-γ appears to play a central role either by inducing Langhans' giant cell formation directly or by enhancing the monocyte-macrophage fusion rates induced by other stimuli. Antibodies against Interferon-γ inhibit giant cell formation *in vitro* as well as *in vivo*.Langhans giant cells are seen in infective granulomatous diseases such as tuberculosis and schistosomiasis or in granulomatous disorders of unknown etiology such as sarcoidosis.[7]

Osteoclasts

Osteoclasts are large multinucleated cells appearing at or near the surface of bone undergoing resorption. Under the light microscope they contain about 10 to 100 nuclei. They are typically located in cavities or pits (Howship's lacunae) on the bone surface, where it participates in the constant process of bone remodelling.[4]

Excessive osteoclast activity in bone resorption has been implicated in pathologic processes such as the advanced stages of multiple myeloma with lytic lesions in bone and postmenopausal osteoporosis.[7]

Histological features of osteoclast:

The osteoclasts are found against the bone surface, occupying hollowed – out depression called Howship's lacunae that they created. Electron microscopically adjacent to the tissue surface, the osteoclast is thrown into a myriad of deep folds/processes that forms a ruffled border. According to Hancox and Boothroyd (1961) and Ham (1974) these processes interdigitate between collagen fibers freed of mineral in the resorptive process. Adjacent to the ruffled border, the osteoclast cytoplasm shows many vacoules, some containing bone salt (apatite) crystals (Cameron and Robinson, 1958), or collagen fibers (Hancox, 1963). Gothlin and Eriksson (1976) showed that the vacoules have the morphological appearance of pinocytotic vesicles. In addition, the osteoclast contains many mitochondria and lysosomes.[4]

There is a clear or sealing zone between the osteoclast and the bone which is undergoing resorption. This clear zone not only attaches the cells to the mineralized surface but also (by sealing the periphery of the ruffled border) isolates a microenvironment between them and the bone surfaces.[7]

Origin of osteoclast:

There is overwhelming evidence that osteoclasts form from mononucleated precursors. A number of possibilities have been put forward for the nature of the precursor cell.[4]

i. Kember (1960), Young (1962) and Owen (1971) suggested that osteoblasts and osteoclasts derive from separate lines of differentiation of a single osteogenic precursor cell.
ii. Tonna (1960-1961), Tonna and Cronkite (1961) observed that osteoblasts may differentiate into osteoclasts.
iii. Rasmussen and Bordier (1974) and Hall (1975) suggested that osteogenic cells may differentiate into osteoclasts and osteoblasts.
iv. Fischman and Hay (1962), Jee and Nolan (1963), Bingham, Brazell and Owen (1969) and Gothlin and Eriksson (1976) described that osteoclast may arise from the fusion of cells of the mononuclear phagocyte system.

There is a controversy whether osteoclasts are derived by fusion of mononuclear macrophages or have a lineage distinct from a macrophage. The calcitonin receptor is the best marker for distinguishing mammalian osteoclasts because this receptor is not expressed on monocyte-macrophage-derived giant cells.[7]

A wide variety of factors can influence osteoclast formation and function. These include systemic hormones, cytokines, and growth factors. It is noteworthy that neither Interleukin-4 (FBGC formation) nor Interferon-g (Langhans giant cell formation) is described as a significant factor in the formation or activation of osteoclasts. These findings suggest that although the colony-forming unit granulocyte-macrophage progenitor is of monocytic lineage, its differentiation does not include expression of Interleukin-4 or Interferon-g receptors or perhaps even a common signal transduction pathway.[7]

Factors regulating osteoclast formation and resorption activity-[7]

Factor	Formation	Resorption
Parathyroid hormone	+	+
Calcitriol	+	+
Prostaglandin E 2	–	–
Interleukin-1	+	+
Macrophage colony - stimulating factor	+	–
Transforming growth factor-a	+	+
Tumor necrosis factor-a and -b	+	+
Interleukin-6	+	+
Interleukin-2	+	?
Calcitonin	–	–
Transforming growth factor-b	–	–
Interferon-g	–	–
Interleukin-4	–	–
Sex steroids	–	–

*Stimulation of osteoclast formation or resorption is denoted by the plus sign (+); inhibition of formation or resorption is denoted by the minus sign (–).

Recent studies demonstrate the ability of Interleukin-1 and TNF-a to induce osteoclast formation and the bone-resorbing activity of osteoclasts. These studies suggest that activated macrophages may facilitate bone resorption by participating in osteoclast formation and activation.[7]

Tumor Giant Cells

These are large cells and posses single huge polymorphic nucleus or two or more nuclei. The nuclei are often hyperchromatic; they stain very darkly and may vary considerably in size and shape. These giant cells are not to be confused with inflammatory Langhans or foreign body giant cells, which posses many small, normal appearing nuclei. The genesis is also different for tumor giant cell and is formed by the division of the nucleus while the body of the cell fails to divide. These giant cells are not derived from the macrophages but from the cells of the tumor, whether connective tissue or epithelial in nature.[8]

Many benign and malignant epithelial and mesenchymal neoplasms contain tumor giant cells (Roizman, 1962). These are usually associated with poorly differentiated tumors and the nuclei of the giant cells resemble those of the mononuclear tumor population.[4]

Nicolson (1976) suggested that tumor cells posses an abnormal surface, this may predispose to fusion in one or several ways. The altered surface charge mosaic may allow close approach of lipid bilayers. Some tumors are associated with passenger viruses, which are known to cause cell fusion.[4]

Reed-Sternberg Cell (R.S. Cell):

Reed-Sternberg cells are tumor giant cells found on light microscopy in biopsies from individuals with Hodgkin's lymphoma and certain other disorders. They are derived from B lymphocytes.[2]

They are named after Dorothy Reed Medenhall (1874-1964) and Carl Sternberg (1872-1935), who provided the first definitive microscopic descriptions of Hodgkin's disease.[2]

Reed-Sternberg cells (R.S. Cells) are large and are either multinucleated or have a bilobed nucleus (thus resembling an "owl's eye" appearance) with prominent eosinophillic inclusion-like nucleoli. Reed-Sternberg cells are CD30 and CD15 positive, usually negative for CD20 and CD45. The presence of these cells is not pathognomonic for the diagnosis of classical Hodgkin's lymphoma. They can also be found in reactive lymphadenopathy (such as infectious mononucleosis, carbamazepine associated lymphadenopathy) and rarely non-Hodgkin lymphomas.[2]

Variants of Reed-Sternberg Cell-

i. Lacunar Cells- These are characteristic of Nodular Sclerosis Hodgkin's Lymphoma. They possess round or lobulated nuclei, vesicular chromatin, and multiple distinct small to medium–sized nucleoli. The voluminous cytoplasm is pale and retracted and thus the tumor cells lie within lacunae. This diagnostic feature is however an artifact of formalin fixation.[2]

ii. Mononuclear Reed Sternberg Cells- They are identical to R.S. cells except that they possess a single round or oval nucleus. They may be found in the various subtypes of Hodgkin's lymphoma but are rare or absent in Nodular lymphocyte predominant Hodgkin's lymphoma.[2]

iii. Pleomorphic Reed Sternberg Cells- They have large, bizarre, polyploid nuclei typical of Lymphocyte depleted Hodgkin's lymphoma.[2]

iv. Mummified cells- These are large necrobiotic cells in which the nuclear details are no longer discernible and the cytoplasm is deeply eosinophillic.[2]

MISCELLANEOUS GIANT CELLS

Touton Giant Cells:

Touton cells are originally called as xanthelasmatic giant cells. These cells have an abnormal size and a foamy cytoplasm. The multiple nuclei are frequently arranged in a wreath-like fashion. These cells represent aberrant lipid-laden tissue macrophages. The lipid droplets are dissolved and removed during histologic processing.[8]

Touton giant cells are seen in lesions with high lipid content such as fat necrosis, xanthoma, and xanthogranulomas.[8]

Warthin Finkeldey Cells:

In 1931, Warthin and Finkeldey, in two separate publications, reported an unusual finding in patients who had their tonsils removed within 1-5 days of clinical appearance of measles.[80] Tajima and Kudow (1976) showed the presence of these giant multinucleate cells in various organs infected with measles virus. Several subpopulations of such cells exist, depending upon the type of tissue in which they are found. Nozawa et al. (1998) have reported that cells in the germinal centres of lymphoid tissue express B-cell markers. Cells in the interfollicular areas and thymus express T-cell marker.[8]

The occurrence of such cells is not specific for measles but appears to be associated with reactive lymphatic proliferation (Kubota et al., 1988; Delsol et al., 1982; Kjeldsberg and Kim, 1981). Kamel et al. (1992) have reported that Warthin-Finkeldey polykaryocytes studied in three cases of lymphoid proliferations express CD43, CD3 and OPD4, indicating that these cells are multinucleated T-lymphocytes.[8]

Such cells are observed also during HIV infections. Orenstein (1998) has reported that in HIV infections these cells most likely represent a multinucleated form of follicular dendritic cells. Their immunophenotype is CD21(+), CD35(+), S100(+). The cells also express actin bundling protein and vimentin.[8]

Aschoff giant cells:

These are multinucleated cells and have a basophillic cytoplasm. These are derived from macrophages rather than muscle. Aschoff giant cells are formed by the coalescing of large Anitschkow Cells. Anitschkow (or Anichkov) cells are associated with, and pathognomonic for rheumatic heart disease. They are also called caterpillar cells, as these cells have a large amount of clear cytoplasm surrounding a rod-shaped nucleus that to some extent resembles a caterpillar. Anitschkow cells are enlarged macrophages found within granulomas (called Aschoff bodies) associated with the disease.[8]

INCLUSIONS IN GIANT CELLS

A variety of inclusions may be found in granulomas, usually within the cytoplasm of giant cells. They are non-specific findings which may be characteristic of one or another entity but are without diagnostic significance.[8]

Asteroid Bodies:

Asteroid bodies may be seen in the cytoplasm of epithelioid or giant cells in sarcoidosis as eosinophilic, stellate or spider-like inclusions. The radiating filamentous arms contain complex lipoproteins, calcium, phosphorus, silicon, and aluminum. Asteroid bodies are not specific for sarcoidosis and can be seen in numerous other lymphadenopathies such as silicone lymphadenopathy.[8]

Crystalline Inclusions:

These are colorless refractile crystals, composed predominantly of calcium oxalate. They are frequently found in the giant cells of granulomas of sarcoidosis and other diseases. In some cases they may serve as the nidus for deposition of calcium leading to formation of Schaumann (conchoidal) bodies.[8]

Schaumann (Conchoidal) Bodies:

They are large concentric calcifications often containing refractile, calcium oxalate crystals. They are usually intracytoplasmic in nature, but if they are numerous or very large, they may be extruded into the extracellular space.[8]

Hamazaki-Wesenberg (H-W) Bodies:

Hamazaki-Wesenberg (HW) bodies in sarcoid lymph nodes. HW bodies are large and spheroidal in shape with a yellow-brown color. These bodies are strongly acid-fast with Fite staining .

They are oval or spindle-shaped, range up to several microns in size, and appear yellow-brown with H&E stain. The pigment appears to be lipofuscin. Ultrastructural studies have shown that H-W bodies are giant lysosomes and residual bodies. They are acid-fast and stain with silver stains as well as a variety of other stains. When visualized with silver stains H-W bodies can be easily mistaken for budding yeasts due to clustering of individual bodies.[8]

FORMATION OF GIANT CELLS

T.J. Chambers (1978) suggested that it is unlikely that polykaryocytosis results from nuclear division without cytoplasmic separation. Indeed, there is much evidence for all mammalian polykaryons being the result of fusion of mononuclear precursors. The very occasional observation of mitosis in a giant cell probably represents mitosis in a recently incorporated nucleus, initiated preceding fusion.[4]

Mechanism of Cell Fusion:

The current concept of the cell membrane is that it consists of a lipid bilayer in which proteins float with varying degrees of lateral mobility (Singer and Nicolson 1972, Nicolson 1972). Many of these proteins extend right through the bilayer, appearing on both inner and outer surface and since they have lateral mobility in the membrane, there exists a mechanism whereby the cell may alter its surface properties from inside.

Conversely, alterations in the position or properties of surface proteins by environmental agents are reflected on the internal surface of the cell and may allow the cell to recognise environmental stimuli.[4]

Poste and Allison (1971) suggested that fusion of surface membrane is always preceded by cell surface alteration. According to Lucy (1975), the lipid bilayer is an inherently stable structure, and needs to be "conditioned" by some destabilising process or agent before it will fuse with other bilayers. Lawson et al. (1977) presented the evidence that during membrane fusion of degranulating mast cells, fusion takes place between areas of membrane from which proteins are absent.[4]

The mechanism by which these cell surface alterations lead to fusion is largely unknown. Since the lipid bilayers are inherently stable structures, the close approach of cell surfaces beyond the normally observed separation distances must be accompanied by changes in the bilayers which render it unstable.[4]

Calcium is known to be important in maintaining membrane stability (Welis, 1967) and the destabilisation which follows its removal may be the common denominator allowing membrane fusion.[4]

I. Mechanism of fusion of macrophages-

Macrophages can be fused either with other macrophages or other cell types to form giant cell in vivo (Gordon and Cohn, 1970). Three suggestions have been put forward to account for macrophage fusion in vivo.[4]

a) Fusion mediated by the immune system
b) Fusion resulting from the recognition of an abnormal macrophage surface by young macrophages
c) Fusion as a result of endocytic activity

a) Fusion mediated by the immune system:

Macrophage polykaryons are commonly found in areas containing poorly removable foreign material. Frequently the foreign material is antigenic (fungi, tuberculosis, etc.). According to Willoughby and Ryan (1970) even when the foreign material itself has no antigenicity (e.g. glass) it is probable that the inflammatory process itself produces antigens. Galindo (1972), Parks and Weiser (1975) suggested that the immune system is responsible for macrophage fusion. It is suggested that the phagocytosing macrophages fuse under the influence of lymphokines. Membrane changes associated with phagocytosis may facilitate the adherence and fusion of macrophages to initiate the formation of giant cells.[4]

b) Fusion resulting from the recognition of an abnormal macrophage surface by young macrophages:

Mariano and Spector showed that enclosing a population of macrophages in diffusion chambers *in vivo* prevented giant cell formation. On leaving the chambers open, however, they found that fresh incoming macrophages fused with those already inside the chamber to form giant cells. They also showed that while enclosed in the chamber, macrophages underwent mitosis which revealed many chromosomal abnormalities. They suggested that the chromosome abnormalities lead to the formation of an abnormal cell surface on the ageing population which is recognised by fresh incoming cells and leads to fusion.[4]

Chambers (1977) tested this hypothesis by exposing xenogeneic macrophages, and macrophages cultured in inflammatory exudates, to fresh macrophages. No fusion was observed between the two populations.[4]

c) Fusion as a result of endocytic activity:

Attachment of any of a variety of substances to the macrophage surface is followed by the formation of endosome margins, which then approach each other and fuse to complete endosome formation. Chambers (1977) suggested that if material is attached to the surface of two macrophages, each macrophage would form endosome margins. The margins of one macrophage would then meet the phagosome margins of the other, and fusion may result between the margins of the two cells, thus resulting in cell fusion.4

II. The formation of polykaryons induced by viruses:

Many cell types can be fused by a wide variety of viruses *in vitro*. Poste (1972) suggested that fusion may be achieved by large doses of inactivated virus or by much smaller doses of infective virus.[4]

With inactivated virus there appears to be a direct interaction between the viral envelope and the cell surface. The viral envelope attaches, leads to a reduction in cell coat thickness, and fuses with the cell membrane. Cell fusion results if the virus is in contact with more than one cell. Antigens from the viral envelope become incorporated into the polykaryon membrane (Heine and Schnaitman, 1971), showing that fusion results from the viral envelope forming a "bridge" between two cells, which subsequently enlarges to complete cell fusion (Poste).[4]

Live virus can cause cell fusion in the same way at high doses, but when the proportion of viruses in relation to cells is low, virus must penetrate a cell and lead to fusion following the appearance of virally coded proteins on the cell surface. The infected cell thus has a surface modified by viral proteins, and this leads to fusion with adjacent uninfected cells. Fusion extends in a plaque to form an expanding syncytium.[4]

Multinucleated cells are seen in man in association with infection by a variety of viruses. In herpes zoster and herpes simplex infections characteristic polykaryons appear (Tzanck and Aron-Brunetiere, 1949). Measles produces Warthin-Finkeldey multinucleate cells in infected lymphoid tissue and in the alveolar epithelium in giant cell pneumonia (Sherman and Ruckle, 1958; Enders et a.l, 1958).[4]

In conclusion, it can be stated that in general cell fusion results from an alteration of the cell surface which allows close membrane approach, followed by the establishment of continuity between the apposed lipid bilayers. The bridge then formed enlarges and nuclei find themselves sharing the same cytoplasmic mass.[4]

CHAPTER 1

GIANT CELL LESIONS

Giant cell lesions of the maxillofacial skeleton and other bones are a controversial matter and uncertainty still exists regarding their basic pathology and biologic behaviour. Fifty years ago, giant cell lesions of the jaws were generally diagnosed as giant cell tumors, and these lesions were widely considered to be similar to those that occurred in the extragnathic skeleton.[10]

Jaffe (1953) reclassified the giant cell lesions of bone and introduced the term giant cell reparative granuloma of jaw bones. This term has the advantage of conveying that the lesion is not a neoplasm. Instead it represents a local reparative reaction. The giant cells found in this lesion are not elements in a tumorous proliferation as they are in giant cell tumour of bone, but they bear a relation to haemorrhage.[11]

However, it has been recognised that the clinical behaviour of a small number of the jaw lesions is inconsistent with the reparative reaction. They tend to behave in a similar way to giant cell tumors of long bones and they are aggressive or recur after treatment. Consequently, several authors felt the need to change the term giant cell reparative granuloma of the jaws to giant cell granuloma or even giant cell lesion.[11]

Whitaker & Waldron (1993) believe that giant cell lesions of the jaws and giant cell tumours of the extragnathic skeleton are not distinct and separate entities but rather represent a continuum of a single disease process modified by age of the patient, location and possibly other factors.[11]

The size, number of nuclei, and the distribution of the multinucleated giant cells have been compared in giant cell lesions and giant cell tumors of the jaw and lesions in other bones. Lucas stated that the giant cells in jaw lesions are often smaller than those in giant cell tumors of long bone. Cells in jaw lesions are unevenly distributed throughout, whereas numerous evenly distributed giant cells are present in practically every field of the giant cell tumors of long bones.[10]

Abrams and Shear (1974) conducted a study on 10 cases of each of the two lesions and confirmed Lucas statement. They concluded that some giant cell lesions of long bones are morphologically indistinguishable from giant cell lesions of the jaws and vice versa. They also suggested that if a giant cell lesion contains giant cells in which the product of length and breadth exceeds 1500 μm^2, the diagnosis of giant cell tumor should be considered. Giant cell lesions are likely to have areas of less than 1500 μm^2.[12]

Whitaker and Waldron (1993) suggested that the giant cell lesions of the jaws represent a spectrum which includes giant cell tumors and giant cell granulomas, and that the features may be modified by local factors.[13]

Giant cell lesions of the jaw occur in two variants: the peripheral and the central (endosteal or intrabony) types. The peripheral giant cell lesion is a solitary soft tissue mass located on the gingiva in dentate persons or alveolar mucosa in edentulous persons. It has been indicated that the ratio between the peripheral and central variants ranges from 3:1 to 4:1. The two variants exhibit identical histological features.[10]

It is widely appreciated however that giant cell lesions of the jaws demonstrate variable clinical behaviour and histopathological features. Although some jaw lesions are slow growing circumscribed processes that respond well to simple curettage, a small number demonstrate aggressive clinical behaviour that is characterized by pain, root resorption, cortical bone destruction and tendency to recur after treatment.[10]

Several studies have been carried out to correlate the various histologic features of the jaw lesions with their clinical behaviour, to determine those that characterise lesions with aggressive behaviour and those that do not. Whitaker & Waldron (1993) reviewed the clinical, radiographic and histopathologic information on 142 cases of central giant cell lesions of the jaws in an effort to determine which of the microscopic features correlate with clinical behaviour.[10]

Chuong et al. (1986) and Ficarra et al. (1987) have suggested on the basis of clinical and radiologic consideration that the jaw lesions can be separated into aggressive and nonaggressive types.[10]

Chuong et al. (1986) defined nonaggressive lesion as those characterized by the absence of or minimal symptoms, slow growth, the absence of root resorption or cortical perforation and a low recurrence rate. The aggressive lesion is characterized by pain, paresthesia, cortical perforation and root resorption.[10]

Whitaker & Waldron (1993) found that an even distribution of giant cells and recognisable mitotic figures occurred in a high proportion of recurrent lesions, as compared with the non-recurrent ones, while the presence of osteoid within the lesional tissue was found in a high proportion of non-recurrent lesions. Several studies on giant cell lesions have reported recurrences with rates varying between 11% and 35%.[10]

According to Whitaker and Waldron, the age of the patient at the time of initial treatment seems to be a factor in the frequency of recurrence. The mean age for patients who demonstrated one or more recurrence was 20 years, whereas the mean age of the patients who did not show recurrence was 28 years. The lesions larger than 3.0 cm at their greatest diameter were more likely to recur than smaller ones.[10]

In the giant cell lesions like Hodgkin's lymphoma, peripheral and central giant cell granulomas and giant cell tumor the multinucleated giant cells are found to be pathognomonic.[4]

In lesions like tuberculosis, HIV infections, measles, xanthoma the multinucleated giant cells are characteristic but are not pathognomonic. In xanthoma, the giant cells are called as Touton giant cell, which are fused foam cells. Its peripheral cytoplasm has a foamy and vacuolated appearance and nuclei surround a central area of clear eosinophillic cytoplasm.

Lesions like fungal infections, syphilis, foreign body reactions, ossifying fibroma, paget's disease, wegener's granulomatosis, fibrous dysplasia, leprosy, Heerfordt's syndrome, odontogenic giant cell fibroma are also associated with the presence of multinucleated giant cells.

Multinucleated cells are seen in man in association with infection by a variety of viruses. Tzanck and Aron-Brunetiere (1949) described the appearance of characteristic polykaryons in herpes zoster and herpes simplex infections. Measles produces Warthin-Finkeldey multinucleate cells in infected lymphoid tissue and in the alveolar epithelium in giant cell pneumonia (Sherman and Ruckle, 1958; Enders et al., 1958).[4]

Biologically, giant cell lesions are characterised by bone resorption. Most of the lesions produce quite well demarcated radiolucencies, while others are widely osteolytic and behave in a locally aggressive manner. Studies of giant cells by Athanasou et al. (1985), Flanagan et al. (1988), and Bonetti et al. (1990) have shown that the giant cells have phenotypic and functional characteristic consistent with osteoclast. Thus, they appear to be an activation of osteoclast formation and activity resulting in bone resorption.[13]

There is considerable doubt concerning the neoplastic nature of multinucleated giant cells in giant cell lesions. They may simply represent a reaction to the mononuclear stroma and may have many of the characteristics of osteoclast. The giant cell lesions associated with the fibro osseous disease of the jaws may be a reaction to a stromal change with in the original lesion.[13]

CLASSIFICATION OF GIANT CELL LESIONS

Based on histological features of the lesions and the presence of giant cells, Chattopadhya (1995) suggested a working classification of giant cell lesions of oral cavity.[14]

1. **Lesions where giant cell in the concerned background are pathognomonic**
   a. Hodgkin's lymphoma
   b. Peripheral or Central giant cell granuloma
   c. Giant cell fibroma
2. **Lesions where giant cells are characteristics**
   a. Tuberculosis
   b. Herpes simplex virus infection

c. Measles

d. Xanthoma

3. Lesions associated with presence of giant cell

Orofacial granulomatosis	Ossifying fibroma
Fungal infections	Aneurysmal bone cyst
Foreign body reaction	Paget's disease
Neoplasm	Wegner's granulomatosis
Fibrous dysplasia	Syphilis
Cherubism	Leprosy
Actinomycosis	Odontogenic giant cell fibroma
Diffuse sclerozing osteomyelitis	Fibromatosis
Heerfordt's syndrome	

Working Classification of Giant Cell Lesions as proposed by Dr. R.V.Subramaniyam-

I. Physiological conditions:

1. Resorption of deciduous teeth
2. Healing of extraction socket
3. Orthodontic tooth movement

II. Infections:

1. Bacterial: eg Tuberculosis, Syphilis, Leprosy, Osteomyelitis
2. Viral: eg Herpes simplex, Herpes zoster, CMV infection
3. Fungal: eg Histoplasmosis, Mucormycosis, Aspergillosis, Cryptococcosis
4. Protozoal: eg Leishmaniasis
5. Chlamydial: Lymphogranuloma venerum

III. Non- infective granuloma:

1. Midline lethal granuloma
2. Wegener's granulomatosis

3. Plasma cell granuloma
4. Sarcoidosis
5. Chelitis granulomatosa

IV. Periodontal Conditions:

Periodontitis, periapical cyst, periapical granuloma, chronic periapical abscess

V. Non- neoplastic growths:

A. Soft tissue	**B. Bone**
• Peripheral giant cell granuloma	• OsteomalaciaCentral giant cell granuloma
• Giant cell fibroma	• OsteomalaciaBrown tumor of hyperparathyroidism
• Pseudosarcomatous fascitis	• OsteomalaciaFibrous dysplasia
• Epulis fissuratum	• OsteomalaciaPaget's disease
• Traumatic granuloma	• OsteomalaciaCherubism
	• Osteomalacia

VI. Cysts & Neoplasm

Cyst: Aneurysmal bone cyst, Calcifying epithelial odontogenic cyst, Solitary bone cyst

Benign neoplasm: Giant cell tumor, Osteoid osteoma, Osteoblastoma, Central hemangioma

VII. Miscellaneous

1. Internal resorption
2. External resorption
3. Massive osteolysis
4. Spindle &/ Epitheloid cell nevus

* For the description of giant cell lesions, we are following Dr. R.V. Subramaniyam's classification.

CHAPTER 2
RESORPTION OF TEETH

Physiological condition:

The exfoliation of deciduous teeth is a physiologic phenomenon and result in the elimination of the deciduous dentition.

The permanent incisors and canines develop lingually to the deciduous teeth and erupt in an occlusal and vestibular direction. Resorption of deciduous tooth roots occurs on the lingual surface, and these teeth are shed with much of their pulp chamber intact. Permanent premolars develop between the divergent roots of deciduous molars and erupt in an occlusal direction. Hence, the resorption of interradicular dentin takes place with some resorption of the pulp chamber, coronal dentin and sometimes enamel.[15]

Histology of shedding:

The cells responsible for the removal of dental hard tissue are identical to osteoclasts and are called odontoclasts. Odontoclasts are readily identifiable in the light microscope as large, multinucleated cells occupying resorption bays on the surface of a dental hard tissue. Their cytoplasm is vacuolated, and the surface of the cell adjacent to the resorbing hard tissue forms a "brush" border. The brush border is resolved as a ruffled border produced by extensive folding of the cell membrane into a series of invaginations 2-3 μm deep, with mineral crystallites within the depth of the invaginations. The cytoplasm of the odontoclast is characterized by an exceptionally high content of mitochondria and many vacoules, which are especially concentrated adjacent to ruffled border. Acid phosphatase activity occurs within these vacoules. Histochemically, a characteristic feature of the odontoclast is a high level of activity of the enzyme acid phosphatase.[15]

Odontoclasts probably have the same origin as osteoclasts. Odontoclasts are derived from the monocyte and migrate from blood vessels to the resorption site, where they fuse to form the characteristic multinucleated odontoclast with a clear attachment zone and ruffled border.[16]

Odontoclasts are most commonly found on surfaces of the roots in relation to the advancing permanent tooth. When root resorption is almost complete, the odontoblasts degenerate and mononuclear cells emerge from pulpal vessels and migrate to the predentin surface, where they fuse with other mononuclear cells to form odontoclasts actively engaged in the removal of predentin and dentin. Just before exfoliation, resorption ceases as the odontoclasts migrate away from the dentin surface, and the remaining pulp cells now deposit cement like tissue on it. The tooth then sheds, with some pulpal tissue intact. During this process, odontoclasts resorb unmineralized dentin.[15]

Non physiological conditions:

Resorption in permanent teeth will occur only under pathologic conditions. This fact appears to be due to the anti-resorptive properties of the precementum covering of the root that protects it in the presence of inflammation.[17]

Since resorption of a tooth may begin either on the external surface (arising due to tissue reaction in the periodonal or pericoronal tissue) or inside the tooth (from a pulpal tissue reaction), the general terms 'external resorption' and 'internal resorption' are used to distinguish between the two types. The chief causes or situations in which resorption may occur are as follows.[18]

1. External resorption
    - (a) Periapical inflammation
    - (b) Reimplantation of teeth
    - (c) Tumors and cysts
    - (d) Excessive mechanical or occlusal forces
    - (e) Impaction of teeth
    - (f) Idiopathic
2. Internal resorption
    - (a) Idiopathic

EXTERNAL RESORPTION

Resorption associated with periapical inflammation:

Resorption of calcified dental tissues occurs in the same fashion as that of bone, and may or may not be associated with the presence of osteoclasts.

A periapical granuloma arising as a result of pulpal infection or trauma occasionally causes subsequent resorption of the root apex if the inflammatory lesion persists for a sufficient period of time. Most teeth involved by a periapical granuloma, however, do not exhibit any significant degree of resorption. The reason for the occasional occurrence is not known. The bone is more readily resorbed than dental tissue is borne out by the fact that bone is always destroyed when a periapical granuloma develops, whereas resorption of the tooth root without loss of bone seldom occurs except at a microscopic level.[18]

Radiographic features:

It appears as a slight raggedness or blunting of the root apex in the early stages, proceeding to a severe loss of tooth substance.

Reimplanted teeth:

The reimplantation or transplantation of teeth almost invariably results in severe resorption of the root. The tooth substance must be considered non-vital tissue. Thus the implanted tooth is analogous to a bone graft which acts only as a temporary scaffold and is ultimately resorbed and replaced.[18]

The tooth root is resorbed and replaced by bone, producing an ankylosis. If the tooth root does not become completely resorbed, the ensuing ankylosis may result in a functional tooth. Many reimplanted teeth, however, exhibit complete resorption of the root and are exfoliated.[19]

Tumors and Cysts:

Both benign and malignant tumors may cause root resorption, although benign lesions are more likely to produce displacement than actual destruction of the tooth. In most cases connective tissue is present between the tumor and the tooth, and it is from this tissue that cells develop, chiefly osteoclasts, which appear to be responsible for the root resorption.

Cysts cause root resorption in a manner similar to resorption caused by benign tumors, that is, chiefly by pressure, although displacement of the tooth is more common than resorption.[18]

Excessive Mechanical or Occlusal Forces:

The usual form of excessive mechanical force with which root resorption may be associated is that applied during orthodontic treatment. Becks reported that systemic disturbances, mainly hypothyroidism, may predispose to root resorption, particularly in the patient receiving orthodontic treatment. However, the influence of systemic factor remains to be confirmed.[18]

The bone undergoes resorption far more readily than cementum when force is exerted upon the tooth by orthodontic appliances or by occlusal trauma. Small lacunae often appear on the surface of the cementum and ultimately extend into the dentin, indicating early tooth resorption. Probably most cases of this minor type of resorption are soon repaired by the deposition of bone or cementum in these ragged lacunae, particularly if the occlusal force or orthodontic pressure is relieved.[18]

From a histological point of view, different degrees of orthodontically-induced inflammatory root resorption severity are determined by the extent to which root tissue is involved. On that basis, 3 different types of orthodontically-induced inflammatory root resorption can be distinguished according to the development following the removal of pathogenic noxa-[20]

— **Surface resorption**- In this process, only the outer cemental layers are resorbed, and they are fully regenerated or remodelled once the etiological factor has been removed.

— **Deep resorption**- In this process, the cementum and the outer layers of dentin are resorbed and usually repaired with cementum material. The final shape of the root after this resorption and formation process may or may not be identical to the original form.

—**Circumferential apical root resorption**- In this process, tridimensional resorption of the hard tissue components of the root apex occurs, and root shortening is evident.

Impacted Teeth:

Teeth that are completely impacted or embedded in bone occasionally will undergo resorption of the crown or of both crown and root. Stafne and Austin reported that teeth that are completely embedded are those most apt to undergo resorption. In a study of 226 embedded teeth in which resorption occurred, they found that 78% of the teeth were in the maxillary arch and that 60% of these maxillary teeth were cuspids. Thus, although maxillary and mandibular third molars far outnumber maxillary cuspids in incidence of impaction, the cuspids undergo resorption more frequently than the third molars. The reason for this is unknown. Impacted supernumerary teeth, particularly mesiodens, also are prone to undergo resorption.[18]

Impacted teeth also may cause resorption of the roots of adjacent teeth without being resorbed themselves. This is particularly common in the case of a horizontally or mesioangularly impacted mandibular third molar impinging on the roots of the second molar.

Idiopathic Resorption:

Many investigators have reported that the roots of permanent teeth may undergo a certain amount of resorption in apparently normal adults without any obvious cause.

Massier and Perreault (1954) in their study observed that the teeth most commonly involved by root resorption were the maxillary bicuspids, while the mandibular incisors and molars exhibited the least resorption.[18]

A rare form of multiple idiopathic root resorptions may occur that involves all or nearly all of the teeth. The resorption may begin at the cemento-enamel junction or nearer to the root apex. This disease has been discussed by Kerr and his associates, who pointed out that these patients, are medically normal and have no past history such as orthodontic treatment or radiation that might explain the phenomenon.[18]

INTERNAL RESORPTION

(Chronic perforating hyperplasia of the pulp, internal granuloma, odontoclastoma, pink tooth of mummery)

Internal resorption is a relatively rare occurrence, and most cases follow injury to pulpal tissues, such as physical trauma or caries-related pulpitis. The resorption can continue as long as vital pulp tissue remains and may result in communication of the pulp with the periodontal ligament.[9]

Sweet has presented a historic review of the internal resorption of teeth, beginning with the first description of the problem by Bell in 1830.[18]

Clinical Features:

Most cases of internal resorption present no early clinical symptoms. The first evidence of the lesion may be the appearance of a pink-hued area on the crown of the tooth, which represents the hyperplastic, vascular pulp tissue filling the resorbed area and showing through the remaining overlying tooth substance.[21]

Roentgenographic features:

The involved tooth exhibits a round or ovoid radiolucent area in the central portion of the tooth, associated with the pulp but not with the external surface of the tooth unless the condition is of such duration that perforation has occurred.[21]

Histological features:

Two main patterns are seen: (1) inflammatory resorption and (2) replacement, or metaplastic absorption. In inflammatory resorption, the resorbed dentin is replaced by inflamed granulation tissue. The resorption continues as long as vital pulp remains. In this pattern the area of destruction usually appears as a uniform, well circumscribed symmetric radiolucent enlargement of the pulp chamber or canal. In replacement resorption, portions of the pulpal dentinal walls are resorbed and replaced with bone or cementum-like bone.[9]

In patients with internal inflammatory resorption, the pulp tissue in the area of destruction is vascular and exhibits increased cellularity and collagenization. Immediately adjacent to the dentinal wall are numerous multinucleated dentinoclasts, which are histologically and functionally identical to osteoclasts. An inflammatory infiltrate characterized by lymphocytes, histiocytes, and polymorphonuclear leukocytes is not uncommon.[21]

In replacement resorption, the normal pulp tissue is replaced by woven bone that fuses with the adjacent dentin.

Treatment and Prognosis:

The treatment of internal and external resorption centres on the removal of all soft tissue from the sites of dental destruction.

CHAPTER 3

TUBERCULOSIS

Tuberculosis is a specific infectious granulomatous disease caused by Mycobacterium tuberculosis. M. tuberculosis infects about one third of the world's population and is the single most important cause of death on earth by infection.[8] It commonly affects lungs but also affects the intestines, meninges, bones, joints, lymph glands, skin, and other tissues of the body. The disease also affects animals like cattle, this is known as Bovine tuberculosis and is sometimes communicated to man.[18]

Etiology:

Two species of Mycobacterium cause tuberculosis: M. tuberculosis and M. bovis. M. tuberculosis is transmitted by inhalation of infective droplets, coughed or sneezed into the air by a patient with tuberculosis. M. bovis is transmitted by milk from diseased cows.

M. avium and M. intercellulare, two closely related mycobacteria, have no virulence in normal hosts but cause disseminated infections in 15-24% of patients with AIDS. Mycobacteria are aerobic, rod-shaped, non spore forming, acid-fast bacilli.[18]

Pathogenesis:

The pathogenicity of M. tuberculosis is related to its ability to escape killing by macrophages and induce delayed type hypersensitivity. This has been attributed to several components of bacterial cell wall-[8]

1. The cord factor, a surface glycolipid that causes M. tuberculosis to grow in serpentine cords.
2. The sulfatides, which are surface glycolipids containing sulphur, prevents fusion of phagosomes of macrophages containing M. tuberculosis with the lysosomes.
3. LAM, a major heteropolysaccharide inhibits macrophage acti-

vation by interferon- gamma. It induces macrophages to secrete TNF-α, which causes fever, weight loss and tissue damage, and IL-10, which suppresses T-cell proliferation.

4. M. tuberculosis heat-shock protein induces auto immune reaction.

The development of cell-mediated or type IV hypersensitivity to the tubercle bacillus probably explains the organism's destructiveness in tissues and also the emergence of resistance to the organisms. On the initial exposure to the organism, non specific inflammatory response develops. Within 2 or 3 weeks, the reaction becomes granulomatous and the centres of granulomas become casseous, forming typical "soft tubercles". The pattern of host response depends on whether the infection represents a primary exposure or secondary reaction.

Clinical Features:

Primary tuberculosis is usually asymptomatic. Occasionally, fever and pleural effusion may occur.

Classically, the lesions of secondary tuberculosis are located in the apex of the lungs but may spread to many different sites by expectorated infected material or through the lymphatic and vascular channels. Typically, patients have a low grade fever, malaise, anorexia, weight loss, and night sweats. With pulmonary progression, a productive cough develops, often with hemoptysis or chest pain. Any organ system may be involved, including the lymphatic system, skin, skeletal system, central nervous system, kidneys and gastrointestinal tract. Involvement of the skin may develop and has been called lupus vulgaris.

Head and neck involvement is not rare. The most common extrapulmonary sites in head and neck are the cervical lymph nodes followed by the larynx and middle ear. Much less common sites include the nasal cavity, nasopharynx, oral cavity, parotid gland, oesophagus and spine.[9]

Oral Manifestations:

Oral lesions of tuberculosis are uncommon.[80] Oral manifestations that usually follow implantation of M. tuberculosis from infected sputum may appear on any mucosal surface. The tongue and the palate are favoured locations. The typical lesion is an indurated, chronic, non healing ulcer that is usually painful.[93] It is frequently found in areas of trauma and may be mistaken clinically for a simple traumatic ulcer or even carcinoma. The causative organism is present in the base of these ulcers, making this a potential infectious hazard to dental personnel. Pharyngeal involvement results in painful ulcers and laryngeal lesions may cause dysphagia and voice changes.[18]

Tuberculosis gingivitis is an unusual form of tuberculosis which may appear as a diffuse, hyperaemic, nodular or papillary proliferation of the gingival tissues.[22]

Tuberculosis may also involve the bone of maxilla or mandible. One common mode of entry of organism is an area of periapical inflammation by way of blood stream, an anachoretic effect or through pulp chamber and root canal of a tooth with an open cavity. The lesion produced is essentially a tuberculous periapical granulomas or tuberculoma.[18]

Tuberculous osteomyelitis of jaws:

Tuberculous involvement of the mandible or maxilla is an occasional complication of pulmonary or disseminated tuberculosis. The organisms enter the bone of the jaws by a hematogenous route and set up a focus within the body of the mandible or maxilla. The bone lesion is that of typical chronic osteomyelitis with a characteristic microscopic feature of tuberculous involvement. Tuberculous osteomyelitis frequently occurs in the later stages of the disease and has an unfavourable prognosis.[18]

Lupus vulgaris:

Primary tuberculosis of the skin or lupus vulgaris may occur in either children or adults and is a notoriously persistent disease. It appears as papular nodules, which frequently ulcerate. These are particularly common on face, but may occur anywhere.[18]

Lupus vulgaris is the most common cutaneous form of TB. It arises when the organisms spread via the lymphatics or blood vessels or is directly inoculated in a patient with basically intact immunity. The over exuberant immune response causes marked tissue destruction.

Initially there are red-brown indurated infiltrated plaques. The plaques spread peripherally, often in bizarre patterns with crusting and ulceration. New satellite nodules may be seen at the periphery. Advanced lupus vulgaris is characterized by massive tissue damage.

Lupus vulgaris is the most common form of TB to involve the oral mucosa, although this phenomenon is still quite rare. It can arise primarily in the mouth or less frequently result from spread to the mouth by perioral lesions.

According to Lloyd and Taylor, the most common oral site is the palate where one sees pale papules or nodules often surrounded by inflammation. The areas then ulcerate. Typically, there are new nonulcerated nodules at the periphery. The base of the ulcer is often granular. Lesions may heal and then break down again with an even more aggressive course.[23]

Scrofula:

Drinking contaminated milk can result in a form of mycobacterial infection known as scrofula. Scrofula exhibits enlargement of the oropharyngeal lymphoid tissues and cervical lymph nodes. On occasion, the involved nodes may develop significant caseous necrosis and form numerous fistulas through the overlying skin.[9]

Histopathology:

The basic microscopic lesion of TB is granulomatous inflammation, in which granulomas show central caseous necrosis. In tissues M. tuberculosis incites a characteristic macrophage response in which focal zones of macrophages become surrounded by lymphocytes and fibroblasts. The macrophages develop an abundant eosinophillic cytoplasm, giving them a superficial resemblance to epithelial cells, in which case they are frequently called epitheloid cells.[22]

Fusion of macrophages results in the appearance of Langhans giant cells, in which nuclei are distributed around the periphery of the cytoplasm. As the granulomas age, central necrosis occurs, which is usually referred to as caseous necrosis because of the gross cheesy texture of these zones.[93] The giant cells are notable in their appearance but are relatively few in number as compared with the mass of histiocyte in the zone of the tubercle. In the ulcer of the oral mucosa the tubercle forms at or close to the oral epithelium, so that the stratified squamous epithelium undergoes necrosis and a large ulceration forms. The floor of the ulcer, as well as the walls presents the characteristic pattern of a tubercle with necrosis, histiocytic and giant cell reaction and lymphocytic infiltration. Because of the ulceration polymorphonuclear leukocytes appear adjacent to the walls of the ulcer.[22]

Diagnosis:

The diagnosis of active infection must be confirmed by demonstration of the organisms by special microbial stains and culture of the infected tissue or sputum. The presence of acid fast bacilli (AFB) in sputum smear is the gold standard for the diagnosis of TB. Imaging techniques like roentgenograph of the affected part like chest and tuberculin test are most useful in supplementing the diagnosis of TB.

Identification of Mycobacteria from respiratory specimens: The demonstration of tubercle bacilli in a respiratory specimen like sputum is a direct evidence of TB. WHO defines any patient whose sputum smear is positive for acid fast bacilli as a case of pulmonary tuberculosis.[18]

Mycobacterial culture:

Conventional mycobacterium culture are done on Lowenstein-Jensen medium, it takes four to six weeks for the growth of M. tuberculosis.

Tuberculin test:

The Manteoux test involves subcutaneous injection of 0.1ml of 5 tuberculin units of purified protein derivative of Seibert stabilized with Tween 80 into the forearm. It is positive if induration is seen after 48-72 hours. The maximum diameter of the induration is measured by palpation and interpreted as follows: more than 15mm or ulceration strongly positive; more than 10mm, positive; 5-9mm, indeterminate; and less than 5mm, negative. A positive reaction indicates that a mycobacterium has replicated in the tissues of the individual at some time but does not indicate an active disease.

Newer methods of diagnosis of TB include radioimmunoassay (RIA), fluorescent antibody test (SAFA) and enzyme linked immunosorbent assay (ELISA), DNA probes and polymerase chain reaction (PCR).[18]

Treatment:

Multiple drug therapy is often recommended as M. tuberculosis mutates and resists single drug therapy. Isoniazid (INH) combined with rifampicin for nine months or INH, rifampicin and pyrazinamide for two months followed by INH and rifampicin for four months. Other drugs used are streptomycin and ethambutol.[18]

CHAPTER 4

SYPHILIS *(LUES)*

Syphilis is a centuries-old infectious disease that has protean clinical features. The name was probably derived from a handsome and wealthy shepherd who was affected by the disease. It is said to have evolved from between 15,000 and 3,000 BC and transported to Asia by Portuguese sailors led by Vasco da Gama. It was an extremely common infection a few decades ago. Widespread use of antibiotics after World War II reduced the incidence of syphilis. However, within the past three decades there has been an astonishing upsurge in the incidence of the disease, much of it in teenagers. Its return is associated with the emerging HIV pandemic.[18]

Syphilis is caused by *'Treponema pallidum',* a spirochete, and is characterized by episodes of active disease interrupted by the period of latency. This is a gram-positive, motile; microaerophilic spirochete and is pathogenic to humans.

Treponema pallidum is acquired by sexual contact with a partner with active lesions, by transfusion of infected blood, or by transplacental inoculation of the foetus by the infected mother.[24]

Classification of syphilis:

Acquired syphilis

- Early infectious syphilis – primary, secondary, early latent (first 2 years of infection)
- Late latent (after 2 years)
- Late syphilis (tertiary) – gummatous, cardiovascular and neurosyphilis[25]

Congenital syphilis

- Early (first 2 years)
- Latent
- Late (including stigmata of infection)[25]

Clinical features:

In the past, there was a male predominance that approached 3.5:1 during certain recording periods. Recently the male-to-female ratio has dropped to approximately 1:1, most likely because of elevated rates of syphilis among women involved in prostitution related to crack cocaine.[9]

Primary syphilis:

Primary syphilis is characterized by the ***chancre*** that develops at the site of inoculation, becoming clinically evident 3 to 90 days after the initial exposure. Although multiple lesions may be seen occasionally, the majority of chancres are solitary. The external genitalia and anus are the most common sites, and the affected area begins as a papular lesion, which develops a central ulceration. Less than 2 % of chancres occur in other locations, but the oral cavity is the most common extragenital site.[26]

Oral lesions are seen most commonly on the lip, but other sites include the tongue, palate, gingiva, and tonsils. The oral lesion appears as a painless, clean-based ulceration or, rarely, as a vascular proliferation resembling a pyogenic granuloma. Regional lymphadenopathy which may be bilateral is seen in most patients. At this time the organism is spreading systemically through the lymphatic channels, setting the stage for future progression. If untreated, the initial lesion heals within 3 to 8 weeks.[9]

Secondary syphilis:

The next stage is known as secondary (disseminated) syphilis and is discovered clinically 4 to 10 weeks after the initial infection. The lesions of secondary syphilis may arise before the primary lesion has resolved completely. During secondary syphilis, systemic symptoms often arise. The most common are painless lymphadenopathy, sore throat, malaise, headache, weight loss, fever, and musculoskeletal pain. A consistent sign is a diffuse, painless, maculopapular cutaneous rash, which is widespread and can even affect the palmar and plantar areas. The rash also may involve the oral cavity and appear as red, maculopapular areas. Although the skin rash may result in areas of scarring and hyperpigmentation or hypopigmentation, it heals without scarring in the vast majority of patients.[27]

In addition, roughly 30% of patients have focal areas of intense exocytosis and spongiosis of the oral mucosa, leading to zones of sensitive whitish mucosa known as ***mucous patches***. Subsequently, superficial epithelial necrosis may occur, leading to sloughing and exposure of the underlying raw connective tissue. These may appear on any mucosal surface but are found commonly on the tongue, lip, buccal mucosa, and palate. Occasionally, papillary lesions that resemble viral papillomas may arise during this time and are known as ***condylomata lata***. In contrast to the isolated chancre noted in the primary stage, multiple lesions are typical of secondary syphilis. Spontaneous resolution usually occurs within 3 to 12 weeks; however, relapses may occur during the next year.[9]

On occasion, especially in the presence of a compromised immune system, secondary syphilis can exhibit an explosive and widespread form known as ***lues maligna***. This form has prodromal symptoms of fever, headache, and myalgia, followed by the formation of necrotic ulcerations, which commonly involve the face and scalp. Oral lesions are present in more than 30% of affected patients. Malaise, pain, and arthralgia are seen occasionally.[26]

Tertiary syphilis:

After the second stage, patients enter a period in which they are free of lesions and symptoms, known as latent syphilis. Syphilis latency is arbitrarily divided into early and late latency stages. The US Centers for Disease Control and Prevention (CDC; Atlanta, GA, USA) consider a duration of infection of up to 1 year as infectious early latency and an infection of >1 year as late latency and no longer contagious. WHO has set the dividing line between these two stages at 2 years.[27]

This period of latency may last from 1 to 30 years; then (in approximately 30% of patients) the third stage, which is known as tertiary syphilis, develops.[28] This stage includes the most serious of all complications. The vascular system can be affected significantly through the effects of the earlier arteritis. Aneurysm of the ascending aorta, left ventricular hypertrophy, and congestive heart failure may occur. Involvement of the central nervous system may result in tabes dorsalis, psychosis, dementia, paresis, and death.[9]

Less significant, but more characteristic, are scattered foci of granulomatous inflammation, which may affect the skin, mucosa, soft tissue, bones, and internal organs. This active site of granulomatous inflammation is known as ***gumma***.[9] It is the result of hypersensitivity reaction between the host and the treponemes or their breakdown products.[18] It appears as an indurated, nodular, or ulcerated lesion that may produce extensive tissue destruction. Intraoral lesions usually affect the palate or tongue. When the palate is involved, the ulceration frequently perforates through to the nasal cavity. The tongue may be involved diffusely with gummata and appear large, lobulated, and irregularly shaped. This lobulated pattern is termed ***interstitial glossitis*** and is thought to be the result of contracture of the lingual musculature after healing of gummas. Diffuse atrophy and loss of the dorsal tongue papillae produce a condition called ***luetic glossitis***. In the past, this form of atrophic glossitis was thought to be precancerous, but several more recent publications dispute this concept.[9]

Congenital (Prenatal) syphilis:

Congenital syphilis is transmitted to the offspring only by an infected mother and is not inherited. Though congenital syphilis is totally preventable, it still continues to be a major problem in many countries. It is recognized that if treatment with antibiotics is begun in infected pregnant women before their fourth month of pregnancy, approximately 95 per cent of the offspring of these mothers will be free of the disease. It is to be noted that not all infected pregnant women deliver children with congenital syphilis. One-third of pregnancies result in abortion or still birth; one-third deliver normal children; and the rest deliver children with congenital syphilis.[18]

Persons with congenital syphilis manifest a great variety of lesions, including frontal bossae, short maxilla, high palatal arch, saddle nose, mulberry molars, Higoumenaki's sign or irregular thickening of the sternoclavicular portion of the clavicle, relative protuberance of mandible, rhagades, and saber shin.[25]

In 1858, Sir Jonathan Hutchinson described the changes found in congenital syphilis and defined the following three pathognomonic diagnostic features known as ***Hutchinson's triad***: Hutchinson's teeth, ocular interstitial keratitis, eighth nerve deafness.[9]

Histopathologic features:

The histopathologic picture of the oral lesions in the syphilitic patient is not specific. During the first two stages, the pattern is similar. The surface epithelium is ulcerated in primary lesions and may be ulcerated or hyperplastic in the secondary stage. The underlying lamina propria may demonstrate an increase in the number of vascular channels, and an intense chronic inflammatory reaction is present. The infiltrate is composed predominantly of lymphocytes and plasma cells and often demonstrates a perivascular pattern. Although the presence of plasma cells within the infiltrate may suggest the diagnosis of syphilis on the skin, their presence in areas of oral ulceration is common place and, therefore, not necessarily of diagnostic significance. The use of special silver impregnation techniques, such as Warthin-Starry or Steiner stains, often shows scattered corkscrew-like spirochetal organisms. In addition, the organism can be detected in tissue through direct fluorescent antibody testing.[9]

Oral tertiary lesions typically exhibit surface ulceration, with peripheral pseudoepitheliomatous hyperplasia. The underlying inflammatory infiltrate usually demonstrates foci of granulomatous inflammation with well-circumscribed collections of histiocytes and multinucleated giant cells. Even with special stains, the organisms are hard to demonstrate in the third stage, and the inflammatory response is thought to be an immune reaction rather than a direct response to T. pallidum.[9]

Diagnosis and Treatment:

Diagnosis is commonly made by serologic testing. The most commonly used screening tests are the Rapid Plasma Reagin (RPR) and the Venereal Disease Research Laboratory (VDRL). These are non-specific, non-treponemal tests that use reagin, cardiolipin-lecithin-cholesterol antigens to test for antibodies against T. pallidum. The most specific serologic tests for syphilis are the fluorescent treponemal antibody absorption test and the microhemagglutination test. These detect antibodies that are produced against treponemal antigens. Dark-field microscopic examination to detect spirochetes is essential in evaluating cutaneous lesions, such as the chancre of primary syphilis or the condylomata lata of secondary syphilis.

Treatment of choice for primary or secondary syphilis is two-team doses of benzathine penicillin G, 2.4 million units intramuscularly, applied one week apart, and for tertiary syphilis three to four doses. Patients who are allergic to penicillin may be treated with either ceftriaxone or tetracycline.[24]

CHAPTER 5

LEPROSY *(HANSEN'S DISEASE)*

Leprosy is a chronic infectious granulomatous disease caused by *Mycobacterium leprae* (M. leprae). It affects mainly the skin and peripheral nerves and also internal organs and mucosa.[29]

Pathogenesis:

An immunologic and epidemiological study suggests most people develop a subclinical infection and very few develop infection. Once infected, both cell mediated and humoral responses are elicited by bacterial antigen DNA glycolipids. Lipoarabinomannan, a component of the cell membrane, induces immune suppression by inhibiting the interferon gamma mediated activation of macrophages.[18]

The bacteria are taken by histiocytes in the skin and Schwann cells in the nerves. This usually results in an inflammatory response involving histiocytes and lymphocytes. It is clinically called as indeterminate type represented as hypopigmented or erythematous macule. The clinical spectrum and ultimate outcome of disease depends upon the intensity of specific cell mediated immunity. Individuals prone to tuberculoid type have an intense cell mediated immune response and low bacillary load, whereas patients with lepromatous type have low specific cell-mediated immune response and a high bacillary load. These two different types are genetically controlled.[18]

Clinical features:

Leprosy manifests in two polar forms, namely, tuberculoid type and lepromatous type. Between these two the borderline and indeterminate forms occur, depending upon the host response.

Currently, leprosy is classified into two separate categories, paucibacillary and multibacillary. Paucibacillary leprosy corresponds closely to the tuberculoid pattern of leprosy and exhibits a small number of well-circumscribed, hypopigmented skin lesions. Nerve involvement usually results in anesthesia of the affected skin, often accompanied by a loss of sweating. Oral lesions are rare in this variant.[9]

Multibacillary leprosy corresponds well to the lepromatous pattern of leprosy and begins slowly with numerous, ill-defined, hypopigmented macules or papules on the skin that, with time, become thickened. The face is a common site of involvement, and the skin enlargements can lead to a distorted facial appearance (***leonine facies***). Hair, including the eyebrows and lashes, often is lost. Nerve involvement leads to a loss of sweating and decreased light touch, pain, and temperature sensors. This sensory loss begins in the extremities and spreads to most of the body. Nasal involvement results in nosebleeds, stuffiness, and a loss of the sense of smell. The hard tissue of the floor, septum, and bridge of the nose may be affected. Collapse of the bridge of the nose is considered pathognomonic.[9]

Oral manifestations:

Oral lesions are uncommon in leprosy but when present occur in patients with the lepromatous form. These lesions are generally asymptomatic ulcers or nodules sometimes rich in M. leprae resembling nonspecific oral lesions.[30]

The locations affected in order of frequency are the hard palate, soft palate, labial maxillary gingiva, tongue, lips, buccal maxillary gingiva, labial mandibular gingiva, and buccal mucosa. Affected soft tissue initially appears as yellowish to red, sessile, firm, enlarging papules that develop ulceration and necrosis, followed by attempted healing by secondary intention. Continuous infection of an area can lead to significant scarring and loss of tissue. Complete loss of the uvula and fixation of the soft palate may occur. The lingual lesions appear primarily in the anterior third and often begin as areas of erosion, which may develop into large nodules. Infection of the lip can result in significant macrocheilia.[31]

Direct infiltration of the inflammatory process associated with lepromatous leprosy can destroy the bone underlying the areas of soft tissue involvement. Often the infection creates a unique pattern of facial destruction that has been termed ***facies leprosa*** and demonstrates a triad of lesions consisting of atrophy of the anterior nasal spine, atrophy of the anterior maxillary alveolar ridge, and endonasal inflammatory changes.[31]

Involvement of the anterior maxilla can result in significant bone erosion, with loss of the teeth in this area. Maxillary involvement in children can affect the developing teeth and produce enamel hypoplasia and short tapering roots. The facial and trigeminal nerves can also be involved with the infectious process.[9]

Histopathologic features:

Biopsy specimens of paucibacillary leprosy typically reveal the tuberculoid pattern that demonstrates granulomatous inflammation with well-formed clusters of epithelioid histiocytes, lymphocytes, and multinucleated giant cells. There is a paucity of organisms; when present, they can be demonstrated only when stained with acid-fast stains, such as the Fite method.

Multibacillary leprosy is associated with lepromatous pattern that demonstrates no well-formed granulomas; the typical finding is sheets of lymphocytes intermixed with vacuolated histiocytes known as lepra cells. Unlike tuberculoid leprosy, an abundance of organisms can be demonstrated with acid-fast stains in the lepromatous variant.[9]

Treatment:

Specific long-term chemotherapy is initiated upon diagnosis. Rifamicin and Dapsone for six months in case of tuberculoid type and Rifamicin and Dapsone along with Clofazimine in case of lepromatous type is usually advocated.[18]

CHAPTER 6

OSTEOMYELITIS

Osteomyelitis is usually defined as the inflammation of the bone and its marrow contents. Changes in the calcified tissue are secondary to inflammation of the soft tissue component of the bone. The term osteomyelitis is reserved for infections which spread through the bone to a larger extent. Though osteomyelitis commonly occurs as a complication of dental sepsis, it is also seen in various other situations.

Predisposing factors include fractures due to trauma and road traffic accidents; gun shot wounds, radiation damage, Paget's disease and osteoporosis. Systemic conditions like malnutrition, acute leukemia, uncontrolled diabetes mellitus, sickle cell anemia and chronic alcoholism may also predispose to osteomyelitis. The disease may be acute, sub acute or chronic and presents a different clinical course, depending upon its nature.[18]

Acute osteomyelitis:

Acute suppurative osteomyelitis of the jaw is serious sequelae of periapical infection. The patient has severe pain, trismus and paresthesia of the lips in case of mandibular involvement and manifests an elevation of temperature with regional lymphadenopathy. The white blood cell count is frequently elevated. The teeth in the area of involvement are loose and sore. Pus may exude from the gingival margin.[22]

Histologic features:

The medullary spaces are filled with exudates. The inflammatory cells are chiefly neutrophils with occasional lymphocytes and plasma cells. The osteoblasts bordering the bony trabeculae are generally destroyed.[97] Bony trabeculae show reduced osteoblastic activity and increased osteoclastic resorption.[22]

Chronic osteomyelitis:

Chronic osteomyelitis may be one of the sequelae of acute osteomyelitis or it may represent a long term, low-grade inflammatory reaction. Mandible is affected more commonly than maxilla. Pain is usually present but varies in intensity. Swelling of the jaw is commonly encountered, loose teeth and sinus tracts are seen less often.[22]

Histological features:

The inflammatory reaction in chronic osteomyelitis varies from very mild to intense. A few chronic inflammatory cells (lymphocyte and plasma cells) are seen in fibrous marrow. Both osteoblastic and osteoclastic activity may be seen, along with irregular bony trabeculae. In advanced cases, necrotic bone (sequestrum) may be present. Reversal lines reflect the waves of deposition and resorption of bone. Inflammatory cells are more numerous and osteoclastic activity is more prominent in advanced cases with respect to milder ones.[22]

Treatment:

The basic treatment of osteomyelitis centers around the selection of appropriate antibiotics and proper timing of surgical intervention.

CHAPTER 7

HERPES SIMPLEX

(Acute herpetic gingivostomatitis, herpes labialis, fever blisters, cold sores)

Herpes simplex, an acute infectious disease, is probably the most common viral disease affecting man, with the exception of viral respiratory infections.[18]

Herpes simplex virus (HSV) is a DNA virus and a member of the human herpes family, known as Herpetoviridae. Herpes simplex virus is composed of double stranded DNA, protein capsid, tegument and lipid envelope, which contains glycoproteins derived from the nuclear membrane of host cells. There are two immunologically different types of HSV: type 1 and type 2. They differ antigenically and biologically, but share 50 percent of the nucleotide sequence. Many types of specific regions exist in both HSV 1 and 2 and are responsible for host immunity. Both are alpha-viruses that are neurotropic, have a rapid replication cycle and broad host and cell range.[32] These subtypes can be distinguished serologically or by restriction endonuclease analysis of the DNA.[33]

The tissues preferentially involved by the herpes simplex virus (HSV), now often referred to as herpes virus hominis, are derived from the ectoderm and consist principally of the skin, mucous membranes, eyes, and the central nervous system. A state of latency and reactivation is common in many viral infections, especially the herpes group. The incubation period is 1-26 days and can occur throughout the year. Transmission is mainly through close contact, kissing, sharing of glasses, cutlery or crockery, etc.[18]

Pathogenesis:

Mucosal surfaces and abraded skin favors the entry of virus and the initiation of replications in the cells of epidermis and dermis. The incubation period appears to range from 2-20 days, with an average of six days before development of lesions.

Initial or primary infection is asymptomatic and occurs commonly in childhood or infancy. Asymptomatic individuals periodically shed infectious HSV in saliva, observed in 2-9% of total cases.[32] Viral shedding is usually greater in immunocompromised patients (approximately 38%) or in those undergoing oral surgery (approximately 20%).[34] Asymptomatic shedding of HSV occurs principally during the prodrome phase of the primary disease.[35]

Herpes Simplex Virus Type 1 infects the oral mucosa by binding to specific cell surface receptors. In the host cell nucleus, the viral genome is replicated, structural proteins synthesized and nucleocapsid assembled. Once inside the cell, replication results in the production of virions that ultimately cause cell death.[32] Following infection and local replication at mucosal surfaces, HSV-1 enters sensory nerve endings and is often transported by retrograde axonal transport to the neuronal cell bodies. Here, a more restricted replication cycle occurs, most often culminating in a latent infection of these neurons. Latency allows the maintainence of the viral genome in a non-pathogenic and non-replicate form and serves as a reservoir for later viral attack of the host. The trigeminal ganglion is the primary site of latency for HSV-1 and the lumbosacral ganglion for HSV-2, in which the virus remains present lifelong.[32]

Though both subtypes produce orofacial and genital lesions, which are clinically indistinguishable, HSV-1 predominantly affects the face, lips, the oral cavity, and upper body skin; and HSV-2 usually affects the genitals and skin of the lower half of the body.[36] Once the primary infection resolves, the virus can no longer be recovered from ganglia but viral DNA can be found in the ganglion cells. Both humoral and cell mediated immunity is responsible for the clinical manifestation, latency, and recurrence of the disease. Immunocompromised individuals, especially with impaired cellular immunity, are more prone for dissemination and recurrence or the primary disease.[18]

Andrews and Carmichael (1930) found that neutralizing antibodies against the herpes simplex virus were present in the circulating blood of most normal adults and persisted throughout life, but that recurrent herpetic lesions frequently developed in these persons.These and other studies have finally led to the established principle that two types of infection with the herpes simplex virus occur. The first is a primary infection in a person who does not have circulating antibodies, and the second is a recurrent infection in persons who have such antibodies. It is impossible to differentiate clinically between the lesions of a primary and a recurrent attack, although the primary infection is accompanied more frequently by severe systemic manifestations and is occasionally fatal. It has been shown, however, that most adults have circulating antibodies in the blood, but have never exhibited a severe primary illness. Thus, it is reasoned, sub-clinical primary infections must be common.[18]

There is an association between HSV-2 and carcinoma of the cervix. However, the link between HSV-1 and oral cancer is less compelling.[22]

Clinical association of HSV-1 infection:

Primary herpetic stomatitis:

Herpetic stomatitis is a common oral disease transmitted by droplet spread or contact with the lesions. It affects children and young adults. It rarely occurs before the age of six months, apparently because of the presence of circulating antibodies in the infant derived from the mother. The disease occurring in children is frequently the primary attack and is characterized by the development of fever, irritability, and headache, pain upon swallowing and regional lymphadenopathy. Within a few days the mouth becomes painful and the gingiva which is intensely inflamed appears erythematous and edematous. The lips, tongue, buccal mucosa, palate, pharynx and tonsils may also be involved. Shortly thereafter yellowish, fluid-filled vesicles develop. These rupture and form shallow, ragged, extremely painful ulcers covered by a gray membrane and surrounded by an erythematous halo. The gingival inflammation precedes the formation of the ulcers by several days.

The ulcers vary considerably in size, ranging from very tiny lesions to lesions measuring several millimeters or even a centimeter in diameter. They heal spontaneously within 7-14 days and leave no scar.[32]

Utilizing culture techniques, August and Nordlund found that the HSV 1 could be isolated from facial, labial, and oral herpetic lesions for a mean duration of three-and-a-half days, with a range of 2-6 days, after the onset of the lesions, while HSV 2 could be isolated from genital lesions for a mean duration of five-and-a-half days, with a range of 2-14 days, after onset. Turner and his colleagues have shown that HSV could survive for two to four hours on environmental surfaces such as cloth and plastic as well as on the skin of the hands contaminated by direct contact with labial or oral lesions.[18]

HSV does not remain latent at the site of the original infection in the skin or oral mucosa. Instead, the virus reaches nerve ganglia supplying the affected areas, presumably along nerve pathways, and remains latent there until reactivated. Unfortunately, this incorporation of viral DNA into host DNA insures a lifelong infection beyond the reach of antibody, cell mediated immune responses or chemotherapy.[37]

Recurrent, or Secondary, Herpetic labialis and Stomatitis:

Recurrent herpetic stomatitis is usually seen in adult patients and manifests itself clinically as an attenuated form of the primary disease. It has been reported by Nahmias and Roizman that between 80 to 100 percent of adults in the lower socioeconomic levels have HSV-1 and/or HSV-2 circulating antibodies, whereas only 30-50 per cent of adults in the higher socioeconomic levels, including medical, dental, and nursing personnel, have such antibodies. Those without antibodies are at higher risk of contact and infection, especially the latter groups because of the nature of their occupation.[18]

The recurrent form of the disease is often associated with trauma, fatigue, menstruation, pregnancy, upper respiratory tract infection, emotional upset, allergy, exposure to sunlight or ultraviolet lamps, or gastrointestinal disturbances. The mechanism through which these various precipitating factors elicit an outbreak of lesions is unknown.[38] The viruses, once they have been introduced into the body, appear to reside dormantly within the regional ganglia, and when reactivation is triggered, spread along the nerves to sites on the oral mucosa and skin where they destroy the epithelial cells and induce the typical inflammatory response with the characteristic lesions of recurrent infection.[32]

Clinical Features:

Recurrent herpes simplex infection may occur at widely varying intervals, ranging from months to years.[8] The lesions may develop either at the site of primary inoculation or in the adjacent area supplied by the involved ganglion. It may develop on the lips or intraorally. In either location, the lesions are frequently preceded by a burning or tingling sensation and a feeling of tautness, swelling or slight soreness at the location in which the vesicles subsequently develop. These vesicles are generally small (1 mm or less in diameter), tend to occur in localized clusters, and may coalesce to form somewhat larger lesions. These gray or white vesicles rupture quickly, leaving a small red ulceration, sometimes with a slight erythematous halo. On the lips, these ruptured vesicles become covered by a brownish crust. The degree of pain present is quite variable.[22]

It has been emphasized by Weathers and Griffin that the recurrent intraoral herpetic lesions almost invariably develop on oral mucosa that is tightly bound to periosteum. Seldom do they occur on mobile mucosa, in contrast to the recurrent aphthous stomatitis which almost invariably occurs only on mobile mucosa. Thus, the most common sites for the recurrent intraoral herpetic lesions are the hard palate and attached gingiva or alveolar ridge. Interestingly, herpes labialis is seldom seen concurrently with intraoral lesions. The lesions gradually heal within 7-10 days and leave no scar.[18]

Histologic Features:

The basic herpetic lesion is quite similar in both the primary and recurrent forms of the disease which differ only in their location and severity. Individual lesions involve the focal death of a group of cells within the spinous layer of the affected epithelium. Liquification degeneration of these cells results in formation of an intraepithelial vesicle, whose central cavity is filled with a proteinaceous fluid. In the mucosa the vesicles tend to rupture early, but in the skin they may persist longer.

The infected cells are swollen and have pale eosinophillic cytoplasm and large vesicular nuclei, described as 'ballooning degeneration". Balloon cells are frequently seen at the edge of the vesicle or may be found floating free in the fluid filled cavity. They are degenerating epithelial cells that become swollen and round because of intracellular edema. When viewed by light microscopy, they appear to have lost their intracellular bridges due to acantholysis.

Cytoplasm of the infected cells forms giant cells. Multinucleated giant cells occasionally are found adjacent to the cavity of the vesicle and are seen more frequently in early lesions. The subjacent connective tissue is usually infiltrated by inflammatory cells.

They are thought to result from the presence of the virus stimulating atypical nuclear proliferation without any equivalent division of cytoplasm in the infected cells. They were first noted by Tzanck and are sometimes referred as Tzanck cells.

ntranuclear inclusion bodies present in the infected epithelial cells are the Lipschutz bodies. These are eosinophilic, ovoid, homogeneous structures within the nucleus, which tend to displace the nucleolus and nuclear chromatin peripherally. The displacement of chromatin often produces a peri-inclusion halo.

When the vesicle ruptures, the surface of the tissue is covered by exudate made up of fibrin, polymorphonuclear leukocytes, and degenerated cells. The lesions heal by peripheral epithelial proliferation.[18]

Diagnosis:

Herpes simplex can be diagnosed both clinically and by laboratory procedures. Scrapings obtained from the base of the lesions are stained with

Wright's and Giemsa stain. Pap stain demonstrates balloon cells, multinucleated giant cells and intranuclear inclusions.

Herpes simplex virus can be demonstrated in the laboratory by isolation of virus in tissue culture or by DNA in the scrapings from lesions. The most sensitive and accurate method for diagnosing these lesions is PCR technique.[34]

Treatment:

Antiviral drugs have significant impact on the course of the disease, if it is diagnosed early. Antibiotic therapy helps in the prevention of secondary infection. Nonsteroidal antiinflammatory drugs and topical anesthetic gel may relieve the discomfort considerably.[39]

HERPES ZOSTER *(Shingles, zona)*

Herpes zoster (shingles) is caused by reactivation of the varicella-zoster virus (VZV) from latency after infection with chickenpox. After acute infection, the virus lies dormant, typically for decades, in the sensory dorsal root ganglia. The cause for VZV reactivation is unclear. However, decline in cell-mediated immunity with age, certain diseases (such as HIV infection), or effects of immunosuppressive therapy are associated with reactivation of the virus. Zoster occurs during the lifetime of 10% to 20% of individuals, and the prevalence of attacks increases with age.[40]

Clinical features:

The disease is most common in adult life and affects males and females with equal frequency. Although rare, it does occur in children.

Initially, the adult patient exhibits fever, general malaise, pain and tenderness along the course of the involved sensory nerves, usually unilaterally. Often the nerve trunk is affected. Within a few days the patient has a linear papular or vesicular eruption of the skin or mucosa supplied by the affected nerves. It is typically unilateral and dermatomic in distribution.

After rupture of the vesicles, healing commences, although secondary infection may intervene and slow the process considerably.[18]

Oral Manifestations:

Herpes zoster may involve the face by infection of the trigeminal nerve. This usually consists of unilateral involvement of skin areas supplied by either the ophthalmic, maxillary or mandibular nerves. The ophthalmic branch is affected several times more frequently than are the second or third divisions. This can lead to blindness secondary to corneal scarring. The involvement of maxillary and mandibular division causes facial and intraoral lesions.

Lesions of the oral mucosa are fairly common, and extremely painful vesicles may be found on the buccal mucosa, tongue, uvula, pharynx, and larynx. These generally rupture to leave areas of erosion. One of the characteristic clinical features of the disease involving the face or oral cavity is the unilaterality of the lesions. Typically, when large, the lesions will extend up to the midline and stop abruptly.

A special form of zoster infection of the geniculate ganglion, with the involvement of the external ear and oral mucosa, has been termed Hunt's syndrome (James Ramsay Hunt's syndrome). The clinical manifestations include facial paralysis as well as pain of the external auditory meatus and pinna of the ear. In addition, vesicular eruptions occur in the oral cavity and oropharynx with hoarseness, tinnitus, vertigo and occasional other disturbances.[18]

When the neuralgia-associated pain persists longer than 3 months after the initial presentation of the acute rash, this is termed postherpetic neuralgia. This occurs in up to 15% of affected patients and at least 50% of patients older than 60 years of age. The pain is described as burning, throbbing, aching, itching, or stabbing, often with flares caused by light stroking of the area or from contact with adjacent clothing. Most of these neuralgias resolve within 1year, with one half of the patients experiencing resolution after 2 months.[9]

Histological features:

Herpes zoster can frequently be recognized by the characteristic distribution of the lesions, although there may be a similarity to the lesions of herpes simplex infection. Skin lesions and oral lesions in particular may be easily identified as viral diseases by cytologic smears and the finding of characteristic multinucleated giant cells (Tzanck test) and intranuclear inclusions.[18]

Infection by the herpes group of virus can be rapidly and reliably diagnosed by a Tzanck test. Ideally, a vesicle less than 3 days old should be obtained since older lesions may get crusted or secondarily infected and the characteristic cytomorphology may no longer be present. The typical features include characteristic multinucleated syncytial giant cells and acantholytic cells. The cells appear as if they have been inflated ("ballooning degeneration") and sometimes may grow tremendously, 60-80 μm in diameter.[41] The giant cells often have a tadpole, bipolar, or irregular teardrop shape with a smooth external contour, in sharp contrast to the jagged configuration of sheets of abraded normal squamous epithelium. Syncytial giant cells contain multiple nuclei (many with 8 or more) that exhibit nuclear molding, so that the nuclei fit together in a jigsaw puzzle like fashion. The nuclei show great variation in shape and size. Intranuclear inclusion bodies surrounded by subtle clear halo are characteristic of herpetic infection, but are often difficult to find.[41]

However, this does not differentiate between herpes zoster and herpes simplex. This can only be done by fluorescent antibody staining techniques, viral culture or serologic diagnosis.

Treatment:

Patients with herpes zoster and intact immune responses have generally been treated empirically. However, it has been shown that oral acyclovir used at high doses can shorten the disease course and reduce post herpetic pain. Analgesics provide only limited relief from pain. Topically applied substance P inhibitor (capsaicin) may provide relief from post herpetic pain. In patients with compromised immune responses, systemically administered acyclovir, vidarabine, or interferon is indicated.[22]

CHAPTER 8

CYTOMEGALOVIRUS

Cytomegalovirus is a member of the herpes family of DNA viruses. Herpes viruses are capable of latency after infection with an acute disease followed by an asymptomatic, quiescent state. Eighty percent of adults have antibodies against CMV. Infection with CMV in most immunocompetent hosts is asymptomatic but can present as mononucleosis like syndrome. A compromise of the host's immune system can lead to reactivation of latent viruses and viral proliferation.[42]

CMV can reside latently in salivary gland cells, endothelium, macrophages, and lymphocytes. Most clinically evident disease is found in neonates or in immunosuppressed adults. In infants, the virus is contracted through the placenta, during delivery, or during breast-feeding. The next peak of transmission occurs during adolescence, predominantly from the exchange of body fluids as this group begins sexual activity. Transmission also has been documented from blood transfusion and organ transplantation.[8] The prevalence of neonatal CMV infection varies from 0.5% to 2.5 %. By the age of 30 years, almost 40% of the population is infected; by the age of 60 years, 80% to 100% are infected. Screening of healthy middle-aged adult blood donors reveals that approximately 50% have been exposed to CMV.[9]

Clinical Features:

At any age, almost 90% of CMV infections are asymptomatic. In clinically evident neonatal infection, the infant appears ill within a few days. Typical features include hepatosplenomegaly, extramedullary cutaneous erythropoiesis, and thrombocytopenia (often with associated petechial hemorrhages). Significant encephalitis frequently leads to severe mental and motor retardation.

Acute adult infection exhibits a clinical pattern that is similar to that of infectious mononucleosis. Most patients have fever, malaise, myalgia, abnormal liver function tests, and atypical peripheral lymphocytes. In contrast to patients with infectious mononucleosis, only about one third of patients with CMV demonstrate pharyngitis and lymphadenopathy. Rarely, immunocompetent patients may show signs of an acute sialadenitis that diffusely involves all of the major and minor salivary glands. In such cases, xerostomia often is noted and the affected glands are painful. Involvement of the major glands usually results in clinically obvious enlargements of the parotid and submandibular glands.

Evident CMV involvement is not unusual in immunocompromised transplant patients. In some cases a temporary mild fever is the only evidence; in others, the infection becomes aggressive and is characterized by significant hepatitis, leukopenia, pneumonitis, and, more rarely, a progressive wasting syndrome.

CMV disease is common in patients with AIDS. CMV chorioretinitis affects almost one third of patients with AIDS and tends to progress rapidly, often resulting in blindness. Bloody diarrhoea from CMV colitis is fairly common but may respond to appropriate antiviral medications.

Although oral lesions from CMV infection have been documented in a number of immunosuppressive conditions, reports of oral involvement by CMV have been increasing since the advent of the AIDS epidemic. Most affected patients have chronic mucosal ulcerations, and CMV changes are found on biopsy. Occasionally, chronic oral ulcerations in immunocompromised patients will demonstrate co-infection (usually CMV combined with HSV).

Neonatal CMV also can produce developmental tooth defects. Examination of patients with a history of neonatal CMV infection revealed tooth defects in 40% of those with symptomatic infections and slightly more than 5% of those with asymptomatic infections. The teeth exhibited diffuse enamel hypoplasia, significant attrition, areas of enamel hypomaturation, and yellow coloration from the underlying dentin.[9]

Histopathologic Features:

Biopsy specimens of intraoral CMV lesions usually demonstrate changes within the vascular endothelial cells. As its name implies, CMV produces enlargement of infected cells. Infected cells exhibit giagantism of both the entire cell and its nucleus. Prominent intranuclear basophilic inclusions spanning half the nuclear diameter are usually set off from the nuclear membrane by a clear halo. Within the cytoplasm of these cells, smaller basophilic inclusions can also be seen. These cells are strikingly enlarged, often to a diameter of 40μm and they show cellular and nuclear polymorphism. These enlarged cells have been called "owl eye" cell.[8]

Gomori's methenamine silver and periodic acid-Schiff (PAS) stains demonstrate the cytoplasmic inclusions but not the intranuclear changes. Salivary ductal epithelium also may be affected and form "owl eye" cells.[43]

Diagnosis:

The diagnosis of CMV is made by considering a combination of the clinical features and by conducting other examinations. Biopsy material can demonstrate cellular changes that suggest infection. Because effective therapies exist for CMV infections in immunocompromised patients, biopsies are recommended for chronic ulcerations that are not responsive to conservative therapy. More specific verification can be made by electron microscopy, detection of viral antigens by immunohistochemistry, in situ hybridization, polymerase chain reaction, demonstration of rising viral antibody titers, or viral culture.[9]

Treatment and Prognosis:

Although most CMV infections resolve spontaneously, therapy often is required in the immunosuppressed patient. Ganciclovir has resolved clinical symptoms in more than 75 % of treated immunocompromised patients. However, the medication must be continued to prevent relapse if the immune dysfunction persists. [9]

CHAPTER 9

MEASLES *(RUBEOLA)*

Measles is an ancient disease but for long time no distinction was made between measles and other exanthematous diseases, including small pox. It was only in 1629 that measles came to be considered as a separate entity. Thomas Sydenham in 1690 gave the first clear and accurate description of measles in the English language.[44]

Measles is an acute, contagious, dermatropic viral infection, primarily affecting children, and occurring many times in epidemic form. It is caused by paramyxovirus belonging to the family paramyxoviridae, which is a RNA virus. Outbreaks are often cyclic in their appearance and are seen commonly at two- or three- year intervals. Spread of the disease occurs by direct contact with an affected person or by droplet infection, the portal of entry is the respiratory tract.[18]

Epidemiology:

Measles is endemic throughout the world and produces epidemics every 2-3 years. Epidemics are usually seen in late winter and early spring, with a peak in April. The disease has maximum incidence in children 1-5 years of age. It is uncommon in the first six months of life due to the presence of maternal antibody. One attack confers solid immunity. Man is the only natural host for measles. [44]

Measles is contagious from first or second day even before the onset of serious illness or appearance of rash. It is transmitted mainly through respiratory secretions and also through direct contact of droplets. The incubation period is generally from 8-12 days. It is mainly transmitted in large families, crowded homes and slums. It is a self limiting disease in healthy immune competent children, but morbidity and mortality is high in malnourished and immunocompromised individuals.[18]

Clinical features:

The disease has an incubation period of 10-12 days and begins with prodromal symptoms of fever, malaise, coryza (running nose), conjunctivitis, and cough. The exanthematous rash follows after a few days and lasts from 4 to 7 days. The face is involved first, with eventual downward spread to the trunk and extremities. Ultimately, a diffuse erythematous maculopapular eruption is formed. The rash clears in a similar downward progression and is replaced by a brown pigmentary staining.

Common complications in young children are otitis pneumonia, persistent bronchitis, and diarrhoea. The less common complication being encephalitis and a delayed complication termed subacute sclerosing panencephalitis (SSPE) which can arise as late as 11 years after the initial infection. It can lead to personality changes, seizures, coma, and death. Measles in immunocompromised patients can be serious, with a high risk of complications and death.[9]

Oral Manifestations:

The oral lesions are prodromal, frequently occurring 2 to 3 days before the cutaneous rash, and are pathognomonic of this disease. These intraoral lesions are called **Koplik's spots**.

Henry Koplik, a New York paediatrician, described these highly characteristic and pathognomonic lesions in 1896. They are tiny 1-2 mm white spots, often with a red rim. These little necrotic areas are usually opposite the molars or grouped around the parotid duct opening. The number of Koplik's spots may range from a few to more than 100.[23]

They are reported to occur in as high as 97% of all patients with measles. Immune reaction to the virus in the endothelial cells of dermal capillaries plays a role in the development of spots. The spots disappear after the onset of rash. These spots usually appear on the buccal mucosa, are small, irregularly shaped flecks which appear as bluish, white specks surrounded by a bright red margin. These macular lesions increase in number rapidly and coalesce to form small patches. Palatal and pharyngeal petechiae, generalised inflammation, congestion, swelling, and focal ulceration of the gingiva, palate and throat may also occur.[18]

Histopathological features:

Initially, Koplik's spots represent areas of focal hyperparakeratosis in which the underlying epithelium exhibits spongiosis, intercellular edema, dyskeratosis, and epithelial syncytial giant cells. The number of nuclei within these giant cells ranges from 3 to over 25. Close examination of the epithelial cells often reveals pink-staining inclusions in the nuclei or less commonly in the cytoplasm. Upon electron microscopy, the inclusions have been shown to represent microtubular aggregates characteristic of the causative paramyxovirus. As the spot ages, the epithelium exhibits heavy exocytosis by neutrophils leading to microabscess formation, epithelial necrosis, and ultimately ulceration.[9]

Examination of hyperplastic lymphoid tissue during the prodormal stage of measles reveals a similar alteration. Within the hyperplastic lymphoid tissue there are numerous multinucleated giant lymphocytes. These multinucleated cells subsequently have been termed **Warthin-Finkeldey giant cells** and were thought for a time to be specific for measles. Since that time, however, similar appearing cells have been noted in a variety of lymphoproliferative disorders such as lymphoma, Kimura's disease, AIDS related lymphoproliferative disease, and lupus erythematosus.[9]

Treatment:

There is no specific treatment for measles. Supportive therapy of bed rest, fluids, adequate diet, and analgesics generally suffices.[22]

CHAPTER 10

FUNGAL INFECTIONS

HISTOPLASMOSIS

Histoplasmosis is a generalized fungus infection caused by the organism *Histoplasma capsulatum*. H. capsulatum is dimorphic, growing as yeast at body temperature in the human host and as a mold in its natural environment. It is usually acquired by inhalation of dust containing spores of the fungus, the contamination probably occurring from excreta of birds.[9]

Clinical features:

The disease is characterized by a chronic low-grade fever, productive cough, splenomegaly, hepatomegaly and lymphadenopathy, since the organisms have a special predilection for the reticuloendothelial system and chiefly involve the spleen, liver, lymph nodes and bone marrow. Anemia and leukopenia also may be present. The infection by this organism may be extremely mild, manifesting only local lesions such as subcutaneous nodules or suppurative arthritis. Histoplasmosis often terminates fatally; particularly the generalized form.[18]

Oral Manifestations:

They appear as nodular, ulcerative or vegetative lesions on the buccal mucosa, gingiva, tongue, palate or lips. The ulcerated areas are usually covered by a nonspecific gray membrane and are indurated.[18]

Histological features:

Histoplasmosis appears basically to be a granulomatous infection which affects chiefly the reticuloendothelial system. Microscopic examination of lesional tissue shows either a diffuse infiltrate of macrophages or, more commonly collection of macrophages organized into granulomas. Multinucleated giant cells are usually seen in association with the granulomatous inflammation.

The causative organism can be identified with some difficulty in the routine hematoxylin and eosin-stained section. Special stains, such as the PAS and Grocott-Gomori methanamine silver methods readily demonstrate the characteristics of *H. capsulatum.*[9]

Treatment:

Acute histoplasmosis is a self limiting process and requires no specific treatment. Chronic histoplasmosis is usually treated by intravenous amphotericin B.

CRYPTOCOCCOSIS *(Torulosis, European blastomycosis)*

Cryptococcosis is a relatively uncommon fungal disease caused by the yeast *Cryptococcus neoformans*. This organism normally causes no problem in immunocompetent people, but it can be devastating to the immunocompromised patient.

The disease is acquired by inhalation of C. neoformans spores into the lungs, resulting in an immediate influx of neutrophils that destroy most of the yeasts. Macrophages soon follow, although resolution of infection in the immunocompetent host ultimately depends on an intact cell-mediated immune system.[9]

Clinical Features:

Primary cryptococcal infection of the lungs is often asymptomatic; however, a mild flu like illness may develop. Patients complain of productive cough, chest pain, fever and malaise. Dissemination of the infection is common in immunocompromised patients and the most frequent site of involvement is the meninges, followed by skin, bone and the prostate gland.

Cryptococcal meningitis is characterized by headache, fever, vomiting and neck stiffness. In many instances, this is the initial sign of the disease. Cutaneous lesions develop in 10% to 20% of patients with disseminated disease. The skin of the head and neck is often involved. The lesions appear as erythematous papules or pustules that may ulcerate, discharging pus like material rich in cryptococcal organisms.[9]

Oral Manifestations:

Although oral lesions are relatively rare, they have been described as craterlike, non healing ulcers that are tender on palpation. Dissemination to salivary gland tissue also has been reported rarely.[18]

Histological features:

The causative organism is gram-positive, budding, yeast-like cell with an extremely thick, gelatinous capsule. The cryptococcus measures 5-20 microns in diameter and in tissue sections, appears as small organisms with a large clear halo, sometimes described as '***tissue microcyst***'. The capsule is colored intensely with the periodic acid-Schiff stain (PAS), and the organisms may be cultured on Sabouraud's glucose agar.

The tissue reaction is essentially a granulomatous one of the tuberculoid type, but focal necrosis is often absent and epitheloid cell proliferation is minimal. Multinucleated giant cells are common, as is a chronic or subacute inflammatory cell infiltrate. The organisms with their characteristic halo are found singly or in groups scattered throughout the granuloma.

Treatment and prognosis:

Amphoterecin B is the drug of choice. The ultimate prognosis of patient is variable and especially dependent upon the sites of involvement.[18]

MUCORMYCOSIS (Zygomycosis, Phycomycosis)

Mucormycosis is an opportunistic, frequently fulminant, fungal infection that is caused by normally saprobic organisms of the class Zygomycetes. These organisms are found throughout the world, growing in their natural state on a variety of decaying organic materials. Numerous spores may be liberated into the air and inhaled by the human host.[45]

Mucormycosis may involve anyone of several areas of the body, but the rhinocerebral form is most relevant to the oral health care provider. Mucormycosis is noted especially in insulin-dependent diabetics who have uncontrolled diabetes and are ketoacidotic. This infection affects immuno-compromised patients, only rarely has mucormycosis been reported in apparently healthy individuals.[9]

Clinical features:

The presenting symptoms of rhinocerebral zygomycosis may be exhibited in several ways. Patients may experience nasal obstruction, bloody nasal discharge, facial pain or headache, facial swelling or cellulitis, and visual disturbances with concurrent proptosis. Symptoms related to cranial nerve involvement (e.g., facial paralysis) are often present. With progression of disease into the cranial vault blindness, lethargy, and seizures may develop, followed by death.

If the maxillary sinus is involved, the initial presentation may be seen as intraoral swelling of the maxillary alveolar process, the palate, or both. If the condition remains untreated, palatal ulceration may evolve, with the surface of the ulcer typically appearing black and necrotic. Massive tissue destruction may result if the condition is not treated.[9]

Histopathologic features:

Histopathologic examination of lesional tissue shows extensive necrosis with numerous large (6 to 30 μm in diameter), branching, nonseptate hyphae at the periphery. The hyphae tend to branch at 90-degree angles. The extensive tissue destruction and necrosis associated with this disease are undoubtedly attributable to the preference of the fungi for invasion of small blood vessels. This disrupts normal blood flow to the tissue, resulting in infarction and necrosis.

A neutrophil infiltrate is typical, and a granulomatous reaction may be observed. This granulomatous infection consists of a chronic exudate of mononuclear cells, histiocytes, epithelioid cells, giant cells and others admixed with connective tissue.[46]

Treatment and Prognosis:

Treatment of mucormycosis consists of radical surgical debridement of the infected, necrotic tissue and systemic administration of high doses of amphotericin B. Despite such therapy, the prognosis is usually poor.[9]

ASPERGILLOSIS

Aspergillosis is a fungal disease that is characterized by noninvasive and invasive forms. Noninvasive aspergillosis usually affects a normal host, appearing either as an allergic reaction or a cluster of fungal hyphae. Localized invasive infection of damaged tissue may be seen in a normal host, but a more extensive invasive infection is often evident in the immunocompromised patient.

Normally, the various species of the aspergillus genus reside worldwide as saprobic organisms in soil, water or decaying organic debris. Resistant spores are released into the air and inhaled by the human host, resulting in opportunistic fungal infection second in frequency only to candidiasis. Interestingly, most species of Aspergillus cannot grow at 37°C; only the pathogenic species have the ability to replicate at body temperature.[47]

The two most commonly encountered species of aspergillus in the medical setting are A. favus and A. fumigatus, with A. fumigatus being responsible for 90% of the cases of aspergillosis. The patient may acquire such infections in the hospital ("nosocomial" infection).[9]

Clinical features:

The clinical manifestations of aspergillosis vary, depending on the host immune status and the presence or absence of tissue damage. In the normal host, the disease may appear as an allergy affecting either the sinuses (allergic fungal sinusitis) or the bronchopulmonary tract. An asthma attack may be triggered by inhalation of spores by a susceptible person. Sometimes a low grade infection becomes established in the maxillary sinus, resulting in a mass of fungal hyphae called an aspergilloma. Occasionally, the mass undergoes dystrophic calcification, producing a radiopaque body called an antrolith within the sinus.[47]

Oral Manifestations:

The presentation that may be encountered by the oral health care provider is aspergillosis after tooth extraction or endodontic treatment, especially in the maxillary posterior segments. Presumably, tissue damage predisposes the sinus to infection, resulting in symptoms of localized pain and tenderness accompanied by nasal discharge. Immunocompromised patients are particularly susceptible to oral aspergillosis, and some investigators have suggested that the portal of entry may be the marginal gingiva and gingival sulcus. Painful gingival ulcerations are initially noted and peripherally the mucosa and soft tissue develops diffuse swelling with a gray or violaceous hue. If the disease is not treated, extensive necrosis, seen clinically as a yellow or black ulcer and facial swelling evolve. Disseminated aspergillosis occurs principally in immunocompromised patients.[47]

Histopathologic features:

Tissue sections of aspergillus lesions show varying numbers of branching, septate hyphae, 3 to 4 μm in diameter. These hyphae show a tendency to branch at an acute angle and to invade adjacent small blood vessels. Occlusion of the vessels often results in the characteristic pattern of necrosis associated with this disease. In the immunocompetent host, a granulomatous inflammatory response in addition to necrosis can be expected. In the immunocompromised patient the inflammatory response is often weak or absent, leading to extensive tissue destruction.[9]

Aspergillus granuloma shows abundant fibrosis, ill-defined epitheloid granuloma, and many foreign body and Langhans-type giant cells. There is no caseation necrosis.[48] Many giant cells show the presence of fungal fragments within their cytoplasm.[49]

Treatment and Prognosis:

Treatment depends on the clinical presentation of aspergillosis. For immunocompetent patients with a noninvasive aspergilloma, surgical debridement is necessary. Patients who have allergic fungal sinusitis are treated with debridement and corticosteroids. For localized invasive aspergillosis in the immunocompetent host, debridement is indicated. This may be combined with either itraconazole or systemic amphotericin B therapy, depending on the severity of the infection.

The prognosis for immunocompromised patients is much worse compared with immunocompetent individuals, particularly if the infection is disseminated.[49]

CHAPTER 11

LEISHMANIASIS

Leishmaniasis is a chronic inflammatory disease of the skin, mucous membrane or viscera caused by obligate intramacrophage protozoan parasite of the genus *Leishmania*, transmitted through the bite of infected sandflies of the genus *Phlebotomus* or *Lutzomyia*.[8]

Etiology and pathogenesis:

Leishmaniasis in human has been classified in three major clinical types: visceral, cutaneous and mucocutaneous. The visceral form of leishmaniasis is caused mainly by L. infantum and L. donovani. Cutaneous leishmaniasis is caused by L. tropica or L. major and the mucocutaneous variant is mainly due to L. braziliensis, but also L. panamensis, L. guyanensis and L. amazonesis.[50]

Clinical features:

Typically, the disease has a long incubation period ranging from few weeks to several years.

Primary cutaneous leishmaniasis usually occurs at the site of the sandfly bite and presents with papulo-nodular, crusted or ulcerated lesions. Mucosal disease affects the upper respiratory tract with a predilection for the nose and larynx. Typically mucosal disease follows an initial cutaneous lesion that has often healed by the time mucosal disease is evident. Visceral leishmaniasis causes fever, hepatosplenomegaly, weight loss, anaemia and hypergammaglobulinaemia.[51]

Oral manifestations:

Oral lesions in leishmaniasis include palatal ulceration, mucosal erythema and fissuring, gingival hypertrophy, papulonodular lesions, sublingual and submandibular lymhadenopathy and tongue swelling with ulceration. Perioral lesions include nodules on the chin, concurrent infections with herpes zoster and cervical lymphadenopathy.

It is well established that leishmaniasis can be a presenting feature of HIV and/or AIDS. Impaired immune system and HIV infection results in increased susceptibility to leishmaniasis.[51]

Histological features:

In the tissue, leishmaniasis is characterized by a subepithelial, non-necrotizing granulomatous inflammatory reaction with lymphocytes, plasma cells and histiocytes. Inclusion within the cytoplasm of histiocytes seen in hematoxylin-eosin staining may suggest the possibility of leishmania (***Donavan's bodies***). The identification of leishmania is possible by Giemsa stain and/or specific antibodies.

In visceral leishmaniaisis parasite invade macrophages throughout the reticuloendothelial system and cause severe systemic disease. Phagocytic cells are enlarged and filled with leishmania, many plasma cells are present and normal architecture of the organ is obscured.

In cutaneous leishmaniasis, the lesion is granulomatous usually with many giant cells and few parasites. In mucocutaneous leishmaniasis, there is a mixed inflammatory infiltrate with parasite containing histiocytes in association with lymphocytes and plasma cells. Later the tissue reaction becomes granulomatous, and the number of parasite declines.[52]

Treatment:

The treatment of choice calls for pentavalent ammonium compounds such as sodium stibogluconate and meglumin antimony. The Centre for Disease Control (CDC) and WHO recommend 20 mg/kg of body weight per day to a maximum of 850 mg/day for a minimum of 20 days and extending for at least 2 weeks after apparent parasitological cure. (WHO, 1990).[52]

LYMPHOGRANULOMA VENEREUM

It is a sexually transmitted disease of men. It is caused by Chlamydia trachomatis (L1, L2, or L3). It is characterized by transient primary cutaneous or mucosal lesion and regional lymphadenitis.[53]

Clinical features:

After an incubation period of 4 to 21 days, a primary lesion develops at the site of infection. The painless, herpetiform lesion, varying 1 to 6 mm in size, usually occurs on the penis, vagina, cervix, but lips, tongue and fingers are other primary sites. Before the primary lesion appears, C. trachomatis is carried in the lymphatics to regional lymph nodes. Here after a latent period of 1 to 4 weeks, the nodes enlarge. Over the next few weeks, the nodes become tender and fluctuant and frequently ulcerate and discharge pus.

Patients with LGV usually present with lymphadenopathy, with or without systemic signs and symptoms, such as fever, chills, myalgias, arthralgias, headache, anorexia and meningismus. Progressive ulceration of the penis, urethra, or scrotum, with fistulas and urethral stricture develop in 5% of men. Chronic ulcers of vulva and smooth, pedunculated, perianal growths are occasional complications.[53]

Histological features:

Primary cutaneous lesion is a superficial ulcer without specific features. The lymph nodes contain characteristic multiple, coalescing abscesses, which have the appearance of granulomas. There are neutrophils and necrotic debris in the centre, surrounded by a zone of palisaded epithelioid cells, macrophages, and occasional giant cells. This zone is surrounded by lymphocytes, plasma cells, and fibrous tissue.[53]

Treatment:

Most infections resolve completely with or without antimicrobial therapy, but there may be serious sequelae.[53]

CHAPTER 12

MIDLINE LETHAL GRANULOMA

(Angiocentric T-Cell Lymphoma; Idiopathic Midline Destructive Disease; Polymorphic Reticulosis; Midline Malignant Reticulosis; Lymphomatoid Granulomatosis; Angiocentric Immunoproliferative Lesion)

The lethal granuloma is a most unusual condition, resembling a serious infection, which has been best described as an idiopathic progressive destruction of the nose, paranasal sinuses, palate, face and pharynx. It was first extensively reviewed by Stewart in 1933. The person afflicted characteristically appears to exhibit complete lack of resistance to the insidious progress of the disease.[18]

The term midline lethal granuloma should be used only as a descriptive designation of a destructive midline condition, and thorough diagnostic evaluation, including biopsy and culture, is necessary to make a definitive diagnosis. Once the other causes of midline destruction have been eliminated, the consensus among most investigators is that this disorder should be classified as a T-cell lymphoma, based on modern cytogenetic, immunologic, and molecular studies

Even though angiocentric T-cell lymphoma often does not have the classic histopathologic features of lymphoma microscopically, it behaves in a malignant fashion and responds to the same treatment to which lymphomas respond.[9]

Clinical Features:

The peculiar granulomatous lesion may begin as a superficial ulceration of the palate or nasal septum, often preceded by a feeling of stuffiness in the nose. It may bear a close clinical resemblance to carcinoma. This prodromal stage, described by Stewart and others, may persist for a month or two to several years. Eventually the ulceration spreads from the palate to the inside of the nose and then to the outside. The palatal, nasal, and malar bones may become involved, undergoing necrosis, and eventually sequestrate. Destruction becomes the prominent feature of the disease and loss of the entire palate is not uncommon. The patient may exhibit purulent discharge from the eyes and nose; perforating sinus tracts may develop, and much of the soft tissue of the face finally may slough away, leaving a direct opening into the nasopharynx and oral cavity. The patient ultimately dies of exhaustion or of hemorrhage if a large blood vessel becomes eroded.[54]

Histological features:

Histopathologic examination of these lesions shows a mixed infiltrate of a variety of inflammatory cells, often arranged around blood vessels (angiocentric). The lesional process appears to invade and destroy the normal tissue in the area. Necrosis is often present in some areas of the lesion, presumably secondary to infiltration of the blood vessels by the tumor cells. Large, angular, lymphocytic cells with an atypical appearance are usually identified as a component of the cellular infiltrate. Immunohistochemical evaluation of this infiltrate often shows a monoclonal T-Iymphocyte proliferation.[55]

A definitive diagnosis of lesion requires the presence of the following histological triad: polymorphic lymphocytic infiltrate, angiitis, granulomatosis (central necrosis).[54]

Treatment and Prognosis:

Without treatment, midline lethal granuloma is a relentlessly progressive, highly destructive process that ultimately leads to the patient's death by secondary infection, massive hemorrhage, or infiltration of vital structures in the area. Lesions that are localized usually respond to radiation therapy. Approximately 4500 cGy is required to control the disease. For patients with more disseminated disease, combination chemotherapy is indicated and a less favorable prognosis can be expected, with 30 % to 50% 5-year survival generally reported.[9]

WEGENER'S GRANULOMATOSIS

Wegener granulomatosis (WG) is a rare multisystem disease characterized by necrotizing granulomatous inflammation of the upper and lower respiratory tracts and kidneys and by necrotizing vasculitis affecting small- and medium-sized vessels. In 1931, Klinger first classified WG as a variant of polyarteritis nodosa. In 1936, Wegener described the disease as a distinct entity with specific clinical and histopathologic criteria.[65]

Etiology:

The specific cause of WG is unknown. Analysis of bronchoalveolar lavage in recently diagnosed patients revealed no evidence of specific bacteria, fungi, or viruses. Although this does not fully rule out an infectious agent as the cause of WG, it does suggest that, if present, the agent is there for a very short period of time and/or cannot be detected by current laboratory techniques.

Some investigators believe that this disease is caused by an abnormal immune reaction secondary to a nonspecific infection or a hypersensitivity reaction to an unknown antigen. A possible hereditary predisposition has been mentioned in some cases.[56]

Clinical features:

Wegener's granulomatosis may occur at any age, from infants to the very elderly, although the majority of cases are in the fourth and fifth decades of life. There is a slight predilection for occurrence in males.[18] Akikusa et al. (2007) in their study observed a significant female predominance, with a male-to-female ratio of 1:4.[57]

The prevalence of the disease has been reported to be 3.0 per 100,000. The disease can involve almost every organ system in the body. With classic Wegener's granulomatosis, patients initially show involvement of the upper and lower respiratory tract; if the condition remains untreated, renal involvement often rapidly develops. Limited Wegener's granulomatosis is diagnosed when there is involvement of the respiratory system without rapid development of renal lesions. One subset of patients exhibit lesions primarily of the skin and mucosa, a condition termed superficial Wegener's granulomatosis. In this form of the disease, systemic involvement develops slowly. These three different clinical patterns highlight the variability of the clinical aggressiveness that can occur in patients with Wegner's granulomatosis.

Purulent nasal discharge, chronic sinus pain, nasal ulceration, congestion and fever are frequent findings from upper respiratory involvement. Persistent otitis media, sore throat, and epistaxis also are reported. With progression, destruction of the nasal septum can result in a saddle nose deformity. Patients with lower respiratory involvement may be asymptomatic, or they may have dry cough, hemoptysis, and dyspnoea or chest pain.

Renal involvement usually occurs late in the disease process and is the most frequent cause of death. The glomerulonephritis result in proteinuria and red blood cell casts. Occasionally, the eyes, ears and skin also are involved.[9]

Oral manifestations:

Involvement of the oral cavity occurs with considerable frequency in WG. However, only rarely are the oral lesions the first manifestation of the disease.[56]

The most characteristic oral manifestation is strawberry gingivitis. This distinctive but uncommon pattern of gingival alteration appears to be an early manifestation of WG and occurs before renal involvement in most cases. The affected gingiva demonstrates a florid and granular hyperplasia. The surface forms numerous short bulbous projections, which are hemorrhagic and friable. The buccal surfaces are affected more frequently, and the alterations are classically confined to the attached gingiva.[9]

The inflammatory process starts in the interdental papilla and spreads rapidly to the periodontal structure and leads to bone loss and tooth mobility.[22]

Oral ulceration also may be a manifestation of WG. These are clinically nonspecific and may occur on any mucosal surface. These are diagnosed at a later stage of the disease. Other less common orofacial manifestations include facial paralysis, labial mucosal nodules, sinusitis related toothache, arthralgia of the TMJ, jaw claudication, palatal ulceration from nasal extension, oral-antral fistulae and poorly healing extraction sites. Enlargement of one or more major salivary glands has been reported. The glandular involvement appears in the early course of the disease.[56]

Histologic features:

Wegener's granulomatosis appears as a pattern of mixed inflammation centered around blood vessels. Involved vessels demonstrate transmural inflammation, often with areas of heavy neutrophillic infiltration, necrosis, and nuclear dust (leukocytoclastic vasculitis). The connective tissue adjacent to the vessel has an inflammatory cellular infiltrate, which contains a variable mixture of histiocytes, lymphocytes, eosinophils, and multinucleated giant cells. Special stains for organism are negative, and no foreign material can be found.

In oral biopsy specimens, the oral epithelium may demonstrate pseudoepitheliomatous hyperplasia and subepithelial abscesses. Because of the paucity of large vessels in many oral mucosal biopsies, vasculitis may be difficult to demonstrate, and the histopathological presentation may be one of ill-defined collections of epitheloid histiocytes intermixed with lymphocytes, eosinophils, and multinucleated giant cells.

The lesions of strawberry gingivitis typically demonstrate prominent vascularity with extensive red blood cell extravasation.[9]

Laboratory findings:

Laboratory findings include an anemia, leukocytosis, elevated sedimentation rate and a hyperglobulinemia. Because of kidney involvement, hematuria is common along with the finding of albumin, casts, and leukocytes in the urine.[58]

Indirect immunofluorescence for serum antibodies directed against cytoplasmic components of neutrophils has been used to support a diagnosis of WG. There are two reaction patterns of these antineutrophil cytoplasm antibodies (ANCA):

1. Perinuclear (p-ANCA)
2. Cytoplasmic (c-ANCA)

Cytoplasmic localization (c-ANCA) is most useful and is present in 90-95% of cases of acute generalized WG. This positivity drops to 60% in early localized form of the disease. When positive, a finding of c-ANCA confirms the diagnosis.[9]

Treatment and prognosis:

The mean survival of untreated patients with disseminated classic WG is 5 months; 80% of the patients die in one year and 90% patients within 2 years. However, the prognosis is better for the limited and superficial forms of the disease.

The drugs of choice are cyclophosphamide and prednisone, but have serious potential side effects. Trimethoprim-sulfamethoxazole has been used successfully in localized cases and when the immunosuppressive regimen has failed. Low dose methotrexate and corticosteroids also have been used in patients whose disease is not immediately life-threatning. New treatment options under study include cyclosporine and intravenous pooled immunoglobulin.[58]

CHAPTER 13

PLASMA CELL GRANULOMA

(Inflammatory Pseudotumors)

Plasma cell granuloma (PCG) is a rare nonneoplastic lesion that was first described in 1973 by Bahadori and Liebow.[18] PCG is a rare soft-tissue tumor that has been reported in almost every site in the body but occurs most commonly in the lung. Plasma cell granuloma is also known as inflammatory myofibroblastic tumor, fibrous histiocytoma, xanthogranuloma, inflammatory pseudotumor, and atypical fibromyxoid tumor because of its variable cellular components.[59]

Clinical features:

There appears to be no sex or age preference. The most frequent clinical picture is a non-specific nasosinusal tumor that grows to a stable state over months or years; it may be painful and may be associated with nasal obstruction, nose bleeding, proptosis, increased lymph nodes, dysphagia or cranial nerve dysfunction. Systemic symptoms are usually not encountered.[59]

Histological features:

PCG was used to be considered a benign disorder. It has been suggested that PCG is the consequence of an abnormality of plasma cell differentiation secondary to chronic infectious or inflammatory processes. It is characterized by cellular proliferation predominantly of polyclonal plasma cells with a variable number of lymphocytes, neutrophils, eosinophils, giant cells, spindle cells and histiocytes, amidst a fibrovascular background. Inflammatory cells are mature and have no cellular atypia or monoclonal proliferation.[59]

Treatment and prognosis:

The most common treatment for PCG is a complete resection; Radiotherapy and/or steroid therapy have sometimes been successfully used to treat patients with non-resectable lesions. With respect to prognosis, PCG seems to be a generally benign, non-recurring condition; nevertheless, local aggressiveness and recurrences may complicate the outcome of the disease.[18]

SARCOIDOSIS

Sarcoidosis is a multisystemic disorder of unknown cause that is characterized by the formation of immune granulomas in involved organs.[86] Jonathan Hutchinson, an English surgeon-dermatologist, reported the first case of sarcoidosis in 1875. The term sarcoidosis was introduced later by Boeck in 1899, which in Greek means, 'flesh-like condition'. Sarcoidosis affects all individuals regardless of race, sex or age.[61]

Etiology and pathogenesis:

Although the etiology of sarcoidosis is unknown, genetic, infectious and environmental factors have been postulated as possible causes. A putative genetic pathogenesis has been suggested due to the presence of familial clusters in sarcoidosis. In addition, positive association with HLA-A1, HLA-B8 and HLA-DR3 has been identified. Studies confirm a genetic predisposition for sarcoidosis and presents evidence for the allelic variation at the HLA-DRB1 locus as a major contributor. The genetic variations that promote susceptibility to the disease may reside in loci that influence the immune response.

Infectious agents such as mycobacterium, propionobacteria, Epstein–Barr virus (EBV), and Human Herpes Virus-8 (HHV-8) have been considered as possible etiological agents but so far the scientific results have been inconsistent and inconclusive. Similarly, environmental factors (wood dust, pollen, clay, mold, silica) and occupational exposure (farmers, fire fighters, military) have been suggested as etiological agents.[61]

Reported evidence indicates an immunological response resulting from one or a combination of factors mentioned above. The T-helper 1 (Th1) lymphocytes play a central role in granuloma formation, which is thought to be the result of deposition of poorly soluble antigenic material in the tissue. This antigenic material is taken up by antigen presenting cells such as macrophages or dendritic cells, which then expose it to T-lymphocytes. In response to these antigens, a local amplification of the cellular immune reaction takes place. In addition, mononuclear phagocytes and other inflammatory cells migrate to the site of the antigenic deposition under the influence of the chemokines and cytokines produced by Th1 cells. This results in the formation of a granuloma.[61]

Clinical features:

Sarcoidosis is usually a self-limiting, benign disease with an insidious onset and protracted course.[93] The disease exhibits a slight female predilection and a bimodal age distribution. The first peak is between the ages of 25 and 35 years and the second peak is at 45 and 65 years. Seasonal variations have been observed worldwide, with the peak incidence observed during late winter and early spring.

Sarcoidosis is a multi organ disorder. The clinical symptoms depend on the ethnicity, chronicity of illness, site and extent of involvement of the organ and activity of the granulomas. One-third of the patients with sarcoidosis can present with non-specific constitutional symptoms such as fever, fatigue, and malaise or weight loss. The most common presentation of sarcoidosis consists of pulmonary infiltration and hilar lymphadenopathy, dermal, and ocular lesions.[61]

Although any organ may be affected, the lungs, lymph nodes, skin, eyes and salivary glands are the predominant sites. Lymphoid tissue is involved in almost all cases. The mediastinal and paratracheal lymph nodes are involved commonly, and chest radiographs frequently reveal bilateral hilar lymphadenopathy. Cutaneous manifestations occur about 25% of the time. These often appear as chronic, violaceous, indurated lesions that are termed **lupus pernio**. Lupus pernio is associated with poor prognosis of sarcoidosis and is associated with more severe pulmonary disease. Scattered, non specific, tender, erythematous nodules, known as erythema nodosum, frequently occur on the lower legs.[62]

Oral manifestations:

Oral involvement in sarcoidosis is uncommon. Oral lesions are the first manifestation of the systemic sarcoidosis in majority of the cases. Schroff (1942) reported the first suspected case of sarcoid granulomas in the oral mucosa, but Poe (1943) reported the first confirmed case of sarcoidosis affecting the oral cavity in the mandible.

The most frequently affected intraoral soft tissue site is the buccal mucosa, followed by gingiva, lips, floor of the mouth, tongue, and palate. The common clinical presentations are localized swelling or nodules, ulcers, gingivitis, gingival hyperplasia and gingival recession. The mucosal lesions may be normal in colour, brownish-red, violaceous, or hyperkeratatotic.

Intraosseous lesions affect either jaw and represent approximately one fourth of all reported intra oral cases. Clinical manifestations when jaw bone is involved are mainly due to the lytic and permeative lesions in the bone and include loose teeth, pain radiating to the ears, nasal obstruction, and non-healing socket.

The disease may also involve the salivary gland. The gland involvement is usually bilateral. Submandibular and sublingual gland involvement is less common than parotid gland involvement. Clinical presentation of sarcoidosis in major salivary glands is usually as painless firm swellings, and fluctuation in the size does not occur during the meal time. Xerostomia may also be present. Other rare but pathognomonic presentation of glandular involvement is Heerfordt syndrome. This syndrome is defined as systemic sarcoidosis characterized by parotitis (usually bilateral), uveitis, and facial nerve paralysis.

It is possible that some of the swellings seen on the mucosa of patients with sarcoidosis are actually expansions of localized involved minor salivary glands.[61]

Histopathological features:

Consistent microscopic findings of sarcoidosis are non-caseating granulomas. The centre of the granulomas usually contains epitheloid macrophages surrounded by a rim of lymphocytes. Occasional multinucleated Langhans type of giant cells is also seen. The giant cells result from the fusion of the epitheloid mononuclear cells and may occasionally contain many inclusion bodies such as **Schumann bodies** or stellate asteroid bodies. Schumann bodies are basophilic, calcified, and laminated bodies derived from lysosomes found in about 48–88% of sarcoidosis patients. **Stellate or asteroid bodies** are found in 2–9% of the cases. They are spiculated in shape and represent entrapped collagen. Some lymph nodes may contain distinctive small yellow brown bodies measuring 1–15 μm in the sub-capsular sinus called **Hamazaki–Wessenberg bodies**. They represent large lysosomes and stain black with methamine silver and red with periodic acid-Schiff stain. The histological findings are not specific to sarcoidosis and may be found in other infectious granulomatous disorders.[61]

Differential diagnosis:

The histologic differential diagnosis include tuberculosis, Crohn's disease, leprosy, cat-scratch disease, fungal infections (blastomycosis, coccidioidomycosis and histoplasmosis), and parasitic diseases such as toxoplasmosis.[22]

Treatment:

Spontaneous resolution occurs in a significant number of patients. Corticosteroids are the drug of choice. Other agents may be used in addition or instead of corticosteroids. Chloroquine has been found to be useful in the management of this disease, either alone or in combination with corticosteroids. Immunosuppressive drugs are used in individuals not responding to corticosteroid management.[63]

CHAPTER 14

CHEILITIS GRANULOMATOSA

(Miescher- Melkersson- Rosenthal syndrome)

Cheilitis granulomatosa is a chronic swelling of the lip due to granulomatous inflammation. Miescher cheilitis is the term used when the granulomatous changes are confined to the lip. Miescher cheilitis is generally regarded as a monosymptomatic form of the Melkersson-Rosenthal syndrome, although the possibility remains that these may be two separate diseases. Melkersson-Rosenthal syndrome is the term used when cheilitis occurs with facial palsy and plicated tongue. The syndrome is occasionally a manifestation of Crohn disease or orofacial granulomatosis.[64]

Clinical features:

Affected patients are found in all age groups, with a median age of 25 years. Cheilitis granulomatosa is episodic with nontender swelling and enlargement of one or both lips. Occasionally, similar swellings involve other areas, including the periocular region. The first episode of edema typically subsides completely in hours or days. After recurrent attacks, swelling may persist and slowly increase in degree, eventually becoming permanent. Recurrences can range from days to years. Attacks sometimes are accompanied by fever and mild constitutional symptoms (e.g. headache, visual disturbance).[65]

The earliest manifestation is sudden diffuse or occasionally nodular swellings of the lip or the face involving (in decreasing order of frequency) the upper lip, the lower lip, and one or both cheeks. The forehead, the eyelids, or one side of the scalp may be involved (less common). The upper lip is involved slightly more often than the lower lip, and it may feel soft, firm, or nodular on palpation. Once chronicity is established, the enlarged lip appears cracked and fissured with reddish brown discoloration and scaling. The fissured lip becomes painful and eventually acquires the consistency of firm rubber. Swelling may regress very slowly after some years. Regional lymph nodes are enlarged (usually minimally) in 50 per cent of patients.

In granulomatous cheilitis, normal lip architecture is eventually altered by the presence of lymphedema and noncaseating granulomas in the lamina propria. The frequency is unknown; the condition is rare. Morbidity depends on whether underlying organic disease, such as Crohn's disease or sarcoidosis, is present. There is no racial and sexual predilection.[18]

Histological features:

The histologic features of cheilitis granulomatosa are rather characteristic, consisting of chronic inflammatory cell infiltrate-particularly peri- and para-vascular aggregations of lymphocytes, plasma cells, and histiocytes and focal noncaseating granuloma formation with epithelioid cells and Langhans type giant cells.[18]

Differential Diagnosis:

Differential diagnosis includes insect bites and sarcoidosis. Serum angiotensin-converting enzyme test, chest radiography or gallium or positron emission tomography (PET) scanning may be performed to help exclude sarcoidosis. Gastrointestinal tract endoscopy and radiography may be used to help exclude Crohn's disease.[18]

Treatment:

Patch tests may be used to help exclude reactions to metals, food additives, or other oral antigens. Some cases may be associated with such sensitivities. If found, avoidance of the implicated allergen is recommended.[97] This condition can be conservatively managed by intralesional corticosteroid injections, nonsteroidal antiinflammatory agents, mast cell stabilizers, Clofazimine and Tetracycline (used for anti-inflammatory activity). Surgery and radiation have been reported to be used.[66]

PERIAPICAL PATHOSIS

Numerous sequelae may follow untreated pulp necrosis and are dependent on the virulence of the microorganisms involved and the integrity of the patients overall defense mechanisms. From its origin in the pulp, the inflammatory process extends into the periapical tissues, where it may present as a granuloma or cyst (if chronic) or an abscess (if acute). Acute exacerbation of a chronic lesion may also be seen. The necrotic pulpal tissue debris, inflammatory cells and bacteria, particularly anaerobes, all serve to stimulate and sustain the periapical inflammatory process.[22]

Periapical Granuloma

Periapical granuloma is a low grade infection and is essentially a localized mass of chronic granulation tissue formed in response to the infection.

The involved tooth is usually nonvital and may be slightly tender to percussion. Percussion may produce a dull sound instead of a normal metallic sound because of the presence of granulation tissue around the root apex. Patients may complain about mild pain on biting or chewing on solid food. In some cases, the tooth feels slightly elongated in its socket. The sensitivity is due to hyperemia, edema and inflammation of the apical periodontal ligament.[18]

Histopathology:

A periapical granuloma is composed of an outer capsule of dense fibrous tissue and a central zone of granulation tissue. The central zone will often contain macrophages with a *foamy* cytoplasm caused by phagocytized cholesterol. Some cholesterol crystals may be present, surrounded by multinucleated giant cells of the foreign body type. Throughout, the soft tissue will be a diffuse infiltrate of lymphocytes and plasma cells. Irregular islands and strands of epithelium are also present which are a result of prolonged, mild stimulation of the *rests of Malassez.*[65]

Periapical Cyst:

A periapical cyst is a common development of longstanding, untreated periapical granuloma. The cyst's epithelial lining is derived from the rests of Malassez. The rests are stimulated to proliferate by the low-grade inflammation of the preceding periapical granuloma.[65]

The majority of cases is asymptomatic and presents no clinical evidence of their presence. They are commonly seen between the ages of 20 and 60 years, but the involvement of deciduous dentition is not uncommon. The most commonly involved teeth are maxillary anteriors. The associated tooth is nonvital or shows deep carious lesion or a restoration which is seldom painful or even sensitive to percussion. The cyst is only infrequently of such a size that it destroys much bone and rarely produces expansion of the cortical plate.[18]

Histopathological features:

The tissue consists of an outer dense fibrous connective tissue capsule that surrounds a central lumen containing a thick, proteinaceous fluid and cellular debris. The lumen is lined by a nonkeratinized, stratified squamous epithelium containing rete pegs that are generally elongated and branched. Collections of cholesterol-laden macrophages are commonly present, particularly in the early stages of cyst development The capsule and the epithelial lining contain a diffuse infiltration of plasma cells and lymphocytes. Cholesterol crystals surrounded by foreign-body giant cells are a common finding. The presence of eosinophilic refractile hyaline bodies, referred to as *Rushton bodies,* is sometimes found in the intermediate cell layer of the epithelium.[65]

Treatment:

If the tooth is restorable, the root canal can be filled, otherwise, the tooth is extracted.[65]

CHAPTER 15

CENTRAL GIANT CELL GRANULOMA

Central giant cell granuloma (CGCG) is an uncommon, benign, proliferative, and non-odontogenic lesion whose etiology is not defined. It was Jaffe who first introduced the term central giant cell reparative granuloma to distinguish this lesion from the giant cell tumor of long bones. However, since a reparative response was quite rare and most of these lesions were found out to be destructive rather than reparative, the word 'reparative' was omitted from that term.[67]

The **World Health Organization** has defined it as "*an intraosseous lesion consisting of cellular fibrous tissue that contains multiple foci of hemorrhage, aggregations of multinucleated giant cells and occasionally trabeculae of woven bone*".[68]

Pathogenesis:

Thought to represent a reparative response to intrabony haemorrhage and inflammation, CGCG was once regarded as a reactive lesion. However, because of its unpredictable and occasionally aggressive behaviour, and because of its possible relationship to the giant cell tumor of long bones, CGCG is best classified as a benign neoplasm.[22]

The histogenesis of CGCG of the jawbones remains controversial, as speculations are still debated regarding the possibility that it represents a reactive, an inflammatory, an infective, or a neoplastic process. Another theory is the vascular hypothesis that suggests that CGCG belongs to the spectrum of mesenchymal proliferative vascular primary jaw lesions. Angiogenesis is a phenomenon modulated by several cytokines and growth factors. Vascular endothelial growth factor (VEGF) and basic fibroblast growth factor (bFGF) are the most potent inducers of angiogenesis and have a synergistic effect. It is produced and released from activated monocytes and macrophages.[69]

Perhaps the most widely held view is that the initial CGCG is an endosteal hemorrhage. In 1962, Kramer stated that if the process is concerned with the repair following hemorrhage, then the repair follows a peculiar pattern complicated by repeated new haemorrhages.[85] El- Labban (1997) studied CGCG and confirmed Kramer's statement. She observed that majority of vessels showed intravascular fibrin thrombi and endothelial cell damage with gaps in the cell walls. Plasma, erythrocytes and fibrin were seen subendothelially. She also noted that one of the gaps in a vessel had been sealed by a giant cell. The author suggested that the presence of the giant cell closed the gap and stopped haemorrhage and the main purpose for the presence of the stromal cells is the repair not only of the hematoma but also of its contributing vessels.[11]

The primary tumor cells of CGCGs are fibroblasts. Secondary cells, which are microscopically the most prominent, are multinucleated giant cells. Accessory cells, seen in considerably smaller numbers, include macrophages, factor XIIIa+ dendrocytes, and endothelial cells. The fibroblasts make up the proliferative component of CGCGs, since they express proteins that are indicative of cells in the cell cycle. Tumor fibroblasts are also believed to be responsible for recruitment and retention of monocytes and subsequently for transformation into multinucleated giant cells.[22]

Clinical features:

The lesion is found predominantly in children and young adults, with more than 60 percent of all cases occurring before the age of 30 years. There is a distinct sex predilection, with a female-to-male ratio of 2:1,[3] which may be explained by recent suggestions of the association between hormonal secretion and the appearance of CGCG in females.[70]

Central giant cell granuloma primarily occurs in the jaws and facial bones; though it also appears in other areas of the body.[67] Lesions occur more frequently in the mandible than in the maxilla. Lesions are more common in the anterior region of the jaws, and mandibular lesions frequently extend across the midline.[68]

In the studies conducted by Stavropoulos F , Katz J (2002) no correlation was found between the size of the lesions, their location and the appearance in different age groups, although the size of the lesion was largest in the younger age group (<30 years). This may be explained by the increased metabolic rate and associated hormonal effects in adolescents; however, scientific evidence to support this hypothesis is not currently available.[22]

Central giant cell granuloma usually is an asymptomatic lesion, which may become evident during routine radiographic examination or as a result of painless but visible expansion of the affected jaw. Cortical bone plates are thinned, but perforation into surrounding soft tissue is rare.[68]

These lesions usually grow slowly, though they occasionally present a high rate of growth and cause some doubts about malignancy.[25] The CGCG are expansive in their growth, but do not invade or grow around nerve trunks. Therefore, the lesions do not cause paresthesia.[71]

Central giant cell granuloma may lead to an expansion in the cortex so long as it grows up. It has been reported the enlarged size of the lesion has caused tooth mobility, tooth displacement, and root resorption. The borders of the lesions may be regular or diffuse.[67]

Since CGCG possesses such different features, Choung et al (1986) and Ficarra et al (1987) have defined the lesion into two types, referring to its clinical and radiographic features-[10]

1. Non aggressive lesions make up most cases, exhibit few or no symptoms, demonstrate slow growth and do not show cortical perforation or root resorption of teeth involved in the lesion.
2. Aggressive lesions are characterized by pain, rapid growth, cortical perforation, and root resorption. They show a marked tendency to recur after treatment, compared with the nonaggressive types.

Studies have failed to identify any biochemical or histologic differences between the aggressive and nonaggressive variants. Most studies have looked for differences in giant cells to make such determinations, but no such differences have been found.[68]

Histological features:

The surgical specimen consists of a soft, spongy, and reddish to brownish friable tissue of varying size. Since the vascular tissue bleeds easily, the specimen is often coated with fresh or coagulated blood.

Histologically, these lesions are characterized by the presence of numerous multinucleated giant cells embedded in a fibrocellular stroma often found adjacent to blood vessel walls.[69] Central giant cell granuloma is made up of a loose fibrillar connective tissue stroma with many interspersed proliferating fibroblasts and small capillaries. The collagen fibres are not usually collected into bundles; however, groups of fibres will often present a whorled appearance. Multinucleated giant cells are prominent throughout the connective tissue, but not necessarily abundant.

Foci of haemorrhage with hemosiderin pigment and newly formed osteoid or bone are occasionally observed in the stroma.[69] The stromal cells may be of atleast two types: one resembles (myo)fibroblasts, oval or spindle-shaped with a cigar-shaped nucleus exhibiting sparse chromatin; the other resembles macrophages with smaller round nuclei exhibiting dense chromatin. The stromal cells project between the giant cells in swirls, with herringbone and storiform focal patterns.

The aggregations of giant cells show great variation in size, morphology, and the number of the nuclei. Morphologically, the giant cells are of foreign body type or osteoclast-like. The stainability of the cytoplasm varies from light basophilia to marked eosinophilia; variations may occur within the same giant cell. Some cells may contain big, ovoid and lightly stained nucleus with prominent nucleoli and sparse chromatin. Other cells contain small, darkly stained nuclei of irregular shape. Cytoplasmic vacoules of different sizes containing erythrocytes, iron-positive hemosiderin granules, and leukocytes are frequently found. Mitotic figures are rarely present. In many instances, the giant cells show a definite relationship to vascular channels. The function of multinucleated giant cells that typify these lesions is still controversial, although most investigators believe that the origin of these cells is related to the fusion of stromal cells with either macrophages or (myo)fibroblast like cells.[10]

The nature of giant cell is still uncertain, but has been considered as phagocytes, foreign body cells, or osteoclasts. The relationship of giant cell with stromal mononuclear cells (MC) has not been fully elucidated. Furthermore, giant cell may simply represent a reactive component of the lesion and may be present only in response to an unknown stimulus from the stroma.[69]

Studies by Liu B et al. (2003) supported the hypothesis that the osteoclast-like multinucleate giant cells in these lesions may arise from the fusion of the mononuclear component, and that the mononuclear cells may be the osteoclast precursors. Their results suggested that the multinucleate giant cells in CGCG express the characteristic phenotypes of the osteoclasts.[5]

A patchy distribution of cellular elements is one feature that helps differentiate CGCG from true giant-cell tumors, which are more homogenous. The histopathologic findings closely resemble, and may be identical with, those seen in cherubism, the aneurysmal bone cyst and the brown tumor of hyperparathyroidism.[68]

Radiological features:

The radiographic appearance of CGCG is not pathognomonic and specific. It changes with the size of the lesion. Small lesions usually appear to be unilocular radiolucent and deprived of internal bone septa. However, large lesions usually appear to be multilocular radiolucent and wispy like bony septae in this area.[67]

Kaffe et al. (1996) found in their study on 80 cases that 51% of the lesions were multilocular, 44% were unilocular, 5% were not loculated, and 68% of the multilocular lesions were in the mandible. They also determined unilocular lesions had a mean size of 4.05 cm, while multilocular lesions' mean size was 7.38 cm. They established a statistically significant correlation between the locularity of lesions and their size. They also described a correlation between root resorption and gender. Root resorption was observed in 24% male patients and only 6% of female patients.[54]

Differential diagnosis:

The clinical differential diagnosis for a solitary or multilocular CGCG includes ameloblastoma, odontogenic myxoma, and odontogenic keratocyst. For patients in the characteristic young age range for CGCG, ameloblastic fibroma, ossifying fibroma, and adenomatoid odontogenic tumor might be added to this list. The microscopic appearance of GCGC is virtually identical to that of the giant cell lesion associated with hyperparathyroidism. This process must be differentiated on the basis of biochemical tests. Elevated serum levels of parathyroid hormone are indicative of primary hyperparathyroidism.

The giant cell tumor of (long) bone may exhibit histologic features similar to those of CGCG. Some controversy still exists as to whether the benign giant cell tumor of bone and the giant cell granuloma of the jaws represents the same disease or two different disease processes.

The size, number of nuclei, and the distribution of the multinucleated giant cells have been compared in giant cell lesions and giant cell tumors of the jaw and lesions in other bones. Lucas stated that the giant cells in jaw lesions are often smaller than those in giant cell tumors of long bone. Cells in jaw lesions are unevenly distributed throughout, whereas numerous evenly distributed giant cells of long bones are present in practically every field of the neoplasm.[79]

Abrams (1974) conducted a study on 10 cases of each of the two lesions and confirmed Lucas statement. They concluded that some giant cell lesions of long bones are morphologically indistinguishable from giant cell lesions of the jaws and vice versa. They also suggested that if a giant cell lesion contains giant cells in which the product of length and breadth exceeds 1500 μm^2, the diagnosis of giant cell tumor should be considered. Giant cell lesions are likely to have areas of less than 1500 μm^2.[74]

Franklin and his associates were able to confirm only a portion of these findings but, utilizing stereological techniques, did confirm significant differences between giant cells of jaw lesions and of long bone tumors in both nuclear numerical density and mean absolute cell volume. The giant cell tumour of long bones has been recognized recently as an infrequent complication of osteitis deformans (Paget's disease of bone).[60]

Other giant cell-containing look-alikes or entities continuing multinucleated giant cells include aneurysmal bone cyst and cherubism. Diagnosis of aneurysmal bone cyst is made by the identification of sinusoidal blood spaces within the tumor mass. Cherubism is diagnosed on clinical pathologic grounds.[4]

Treatment & prognosis:

Conventional management is by curettage or resection, which may be associated with loss of teeth, or in the younger patient, developing tooth germs. Non-surgical treatment includes systemic calcitonin therapy and intralesional injections with corticosteroids.[80]

CHAPTER 16

PERIPHERAL GIANT CELL GRANULOMA

(Peripheral giant cell epulis, peripheral giant cell reparative granuloma)

Peripheral giant cell granuloma (PGCG) is the most frequent giant cell lesion of the jaws, and originates from the connective tissue of the periosteum or from the periodontal membrane, in response to local irritation or chronic trauma.

Etiology and Pathogenesis:

Peripheral giant cell granuloma (PGCG) is not a true neoplasm but rather a benign hyperplastic reactive lesion caused by local irritation or chronic trauma. The condition has also been referred to as peripheral giant cell tumor, giant cell epulis, reparatory giant cell granuloma and giant cell hyperplasia of the oral mucosa.[77]

Clinical features:

Although the lesion may be found in very young children as well as in dentulous or edentulous elderly person, most patients were in fourth to sixth decades of life and the mean age of patients at the time of diagnosis is typically 38-42 years.

Bodner L et al. (1997) in their study on 79 patients concluded that the ages ranged between 8 to 85 years (average 53 years). The male/female ratio was 1:2.75. 73% PGCG occurred in the mandible, and 27% occurred in the maxilla. The size of the lesion in its largest dimension ranged between 2 and 5 cm (average 3.2 cm). The site of the lesion was within the teeth bearing area even among the edentulous patients. The posterior (premolar and molar) region of the jaw was the most common site of occurrence.

Gandara JM et al. (2002) in their study observed that mean patient age was 50 years (range 13-78 years). They also reported that 61.5% of the patients were women. In 61.5% of the patients the lesion was in the upper jaw; in 54% of the patients the lesion was anterior.

There is no evidence to support any racial predilection for PGCG, and cases have been reported in Asians, Caucasians and Black people.[77]

Pandolfi et al. (1999) studied the potentially aggressive nature of PGCG in the growing child, and demonstrated resorption of adjacent bone and tooth displacement and multiple recurrences.[81]

Peripheral giant cell granulomas are seen exclusively in gingiva, usually between the first permanent molars and the incisors. They presumably arise from periodontal ligament or periosteum and cause, on occasion, resorption of alveolar bone. When this process occurs on the edentulous ridge, a superficial, cup-shaped radiolucency may be seen.

Clinically, PGCG manifests as a firm, soft, bright nodule or as a sessile or pediculate mass. The color can range from dark red to purple or blue, and the surface is occasionally ulcerated. The lesions range in size from small papules to enlarged masses, and are generally soft or rubbery to touch. They are basically asymptomatic, unless they interfere with occlusion, in which case they may ulcerate and become infected.

In the edentulous patient, the lesion may appear sometimes as a vascular, ovoid or fusiform swelling of the crest of the ridge, seldom over 1-2 cm in diameter. Or there may be a granular mass of tissue which seems to be growing from the tissue covering the slope of the ridge. The color of these lesions varies, but is usually similar to that of lesions in dentulous patients. Ulceration is less common in the edentulous situation. A slight predilection for the mandible is observed in most reported series.

Although incipient lesions may bleed and induce minor changes in gingival contour, gradual growth in some cases produces an important tumor mass that adversely affects normal oral function. Pain is not a common characteristic, and lesion growth in most cases is induced by repeated trauma. These are soft tissue lesions that rarely affect the underlying bone, though the latter may suffer erosion.[77]

Histological features:

Histologically, PGCG is described as a non-encapsulated mass of tissue composed of a reticular and fibrillar connective tissue stroma containing abundant young connective tissue cells of ovoid or fusiform shape, and multinucleated giant cells.[74]

The lesion typically contains abundant capillaries, particularly in the more peripheral zones, and giant cells are sometimes identified in the internal wall of these vessels. Hemorrhagic foci are also typical, with the release of hemosiderin pigment and posterior invasion by mononuclear phagocytes and inflammatory cells. The giant cells are immersed within the stromal component of fibroblasts, immature cells and ground substance (collagen fibers, reticulin and ground substance proper) – the composition of which varies according to the evolutive stage of the lesion. Spicules of newly formed osteoid or bone are often found scattered throughout the vascular and cellular fibrous lesion.[82]

The histological study centres on three points: epithelium, connective tissue zone and medullary or core region[73]:

- The lining epithelium corresponds to the squamous structure of the gums, which may suffer ulcerative changes.
- The subepithelial connective tissue zone is composed of connective tissue with abundant small-caliber blood vessels. An acute inflammatory infiltrate is often seen.
- The medullary or core region is where the giant cells are located. These may be of two types:[73]

Type A cells: Polynuclear eosinophilic cells with a diffuse and abundant cytoplasm. The nucleus is prominent, and the chromatin is distributed along the internal membrane.

Type B cells: Cells with a regular and well defined, more chromatic and larger cytoplasm. The nuclei present poorly defined limits and show a central accumulation tendency, with intense hyperchromatism.

A histochemical study of this lesion has been reported by Shklar and Cataldo with distinct differences observed in different multinucleated giant cells with respect to the distribution of tyrosine and sulfhydryl groups.[18]

The origin of the giant cells has never been established. Although their resemblance to osteoclasts is sometimes striking, seldom are they seen carrying out the ascribed normal resorptive function of such cells. Geschickter and Copeland suggested that the giant cells might be derived from proliferating giant cells associated with the resorption of deciduous tooth roots. Thus they suppose the lesion to be concerned with the transition from the deciduous to the permanent dentition. Unfortunately, such association of lesions is present in only a few cases even though the tumor is a rather common one in youngsters. Such a theory would account for the predominance of the lesions anterior to the permanent molars.

There has been considerable support for another theory of origin from endothelial cells of capillaries. There is some basis in fact for such an idea, the chief being the common occurrence of the giant cells within vascular channels, suggesting that they arise here through fusion of endothelial cell. This suggested to earlier workers that the tumor was a malignant metastasizing one, and they applied to it the term 'giant cell sarcoma' or in some cases, 'myeloid sarcoma'.

A recent study of the giant cells in the peripheral giant cell granuloma by electron microscopy has been reported by Sapp. He found that these giant cells ultra structurally contained a sufficient number of features in common with osteoclasts to conclude that they represent a slightly modified form of that cell. In addition, he reported that the stromal cells were structurally compatible with the various stages of differentiating osteoprogenitor cells.[18]

Caravalho et al. (1995) in their study of ultra structure of PGCG revealed three types of mononuclear cells. The first type showed vacoules containing phagocytosed collagen fibrils or membranous debris and morphological characteristics suggesting that these cells are part of the mononuclear phagocytic system. Some of these mononuclear cells presented interdigitated cytoplasmic processes in close association, suggesting fusion to produce giant cells.

Other mononuclear cells were interpreted as stromal fibroblasts and sometimes showed a great number of collagen fibrils in the intercellular space around them. The last type of mononuclear cells corresponds to Langhans cells.

Laboratory studies are generally not necessary. Serum calcium level or a parathyroid hormone assay may be indicated to rule out the rare possibility of brown tumor for lesions that are particularly large and recurrent, may be associated with systemic signs of hyperparathyroidism.[82]

Radiologic features:

The intraoral roentgenogram may or may not exhibit evidence of involvement of the bone underlying the lesion.[97] The X-ray features are nonspecific, with foci of bone metaplasia in some cases. Some patients may present evidence of bone involvement beneath the lesion, in the form of superficial alveolar bone resorption – observable on periapical X-rays. Widening of the periodontal ligament space is often a finding associated to dental mobility, though in some situations it may represent lesion spread around the root. Detailed examination of the zone can reveal small bone spicules extending vertically towards the base of the lesion.

In edentulous areas the peripheral giant cell granuloma characteristically exhibits superficial erosion of the bone with pathognomonic peripheral 'cuffing' of the bone as seen in the roentgenogram. When the tumor occurs in areas in which teeth are present, the roentgenogram may reveal superficial destruction of the alveolar margin or crest of the interdental bone, but this is by no means invariably present.

X-rays are important for determining whether the lesion is of gingival (i.e., peripheral) origin or of bone (central) origin with spread towards the surface.[73]

Differential diagnosis:

A range of disorders should be considered in the differential diagnosis of peripheral granuloma, including pyogenic granuloma, fibrous epulis, peripheral ossifying fibroma, inflammatory fibrous hyperplasia, peripheral odontogenic fibroma, hemangioma cavernosum and papilloma. The histological study of the resected tissue establishes the definitive diagnosis.

From the histopathological perspective, the principal differential diagnosis is established with central giant cell granuloma, though the clinical and radiological findings offer a clear and conclusive distinction between central and peripheral giant cell granuloma.[73]

Treatment & prognosis:

The treatment of PGCG comprises surgical resection and suppression of the underlying etiologic factors – with elimination of the entire base of the lesion.[23] Conservative excision is typically curative, although the lesion must be completely removed to prevent recurrence. Prognosis is excellent. A recurrence rate of 10-15 per cent has been reported in most series; however, recurrences are typically managed easily with additional surgery.[18]

CHAPTER 17

HYPERPARATHYROIDISM

Hyperparathyroidism is produced by the excess production of parathyroid hormone (PTH) which is normally produced by the parathyroid glands in response to a decrease in serum calcium levels. Rarely, it may be associated with a Noonan-type syndrome, a complex, autosomal dominant inherited trait comprising short stature, unusual facies, mental retardation and cardiac defects. It may be one of the three types – Primary, Secondary or Hereditary.[9]

Primary hyperparathyroidism *(Osteitis fibrosa cystica)* is a condition caused by an overproduction of PTH, in excess of the amount required by the body. It is usually a result of a parathyroid adenoma (80% to 90% of cases) or parathyroid hyperplasia (10% to 15% of cases). Infrequently (in less than *2%* of cases), a parathyroid carcinoma may be the cause of primary hyperparathyroidism.[9]

Characteristic abnormal findings are elevated parathormone level, calcium and phosphatase levels resulting from parathormone stimulation of osteoclast mediated bone resorption, from decreasing calcium excretion in the kidneys and from increased intestinal reabsorption. These elevated levels may be manifested by poor muscle tone and decreased muscular excitability.[18]

Secondary hyperparathyroidism refers to increased PTH secretion as a secondary effect of other disorders, rather than from intrinsic disease of the parathyroids. It develops in response to chronic low levels of serum calcium which is mainly associated with chronic renal disease.

Tertiary hyperparathyroidism refers to hypercalcaemia arising from excessive PTH secretion in the setting of longstanding secondary hyperparathyroidism. Tertiary hyperparathyroidism occurs mainly in patients on dialysis or after renal transplant. It is biochemically similar to primary hyperparathyroidism.[83]

Clinical and Radiographic Features:

Hyperparathyroidism is a rare disease which is said to be three times more common in women. It usually affects middle age but may occur in childhood or in later life. Its incidence increases with age and is greater in postmenopausal women. Early symptoms include fatigue, weakness, nausea, anorexia, arrhythmias, polyurea, thirst, depression and constipation.[84]

Patients may have classic triad of signs and symptoms of hyperparathyroidism, and are described as having "stones, bones, and abdominal groans".

Stones refer to the fact that these patients, particularly those with primary hyperparathyroidism, have a marked tendency to develop renal calculi (kidney stones, nephrolithiasis) because of the elevated serum calcium levels.[22]

Bones refers to a variety of osseous changes that may occur in conjunction with hyperparathyroidism. Generalized loss of the lamina dura surrounding the roots of the teeth is also seen as an early manifestation of the condition. Alterations in trabecular pattern characteristically develop next. A decrease in trabecular density and blurring of the normal trabecular pattern occur; often a "ground glass" appearance results.[9]

With persistent disease, other osseous lesions develop, such as the so-called Brown tumor of hyperparathyroidism. These lesions appear radiographically as well-demarcated unilocular or multilocular radiolucencies. They commonly affect the mandible, clavicles, ribs, and pelvis. They may be solitary but are often multiple, and longstanding lesions may produce significant cortical expansion. The most severe skeletal manifestation of chronic hyperparathyroidism has been called osteitis fibrosa cystica, a condition that develops from the central degeneration and fibrosis of longstanding brown tumors. In patients with secondary hyperparathyroidism caused by end-stage renal disease (renal osteodystrophy), striking enlargement of the jaws has been known to occur and produce a ground-glass radiographic pattern.

Abdominal groan refers to the tendency for the development of duodenal ulcers. In addition, changes in mental status are often seen, ranging from lethargy and weakness to confusion or dementia.[84]

Histopathologic features:

The Brown tumor of hyperparathyroidism derives its name from the color of the tissue specimen, which is usually a dark reddish-brown because of the abundant hemorrhage and hemosiderin deposition within the tumor. This lesion is characterized by a proliferation of exceedingly vascular granulation tissue, which serves as a background for numerous multinucleated osteoclast-type giant cells.

Histologic findings in the bone lesions are not pathognomonic of the disease. Laboratory investigations show increased calcium levels that may exceed upto 16 to 17 mg/dl. Some lesions may also show a proliferative response characterized by arrangement of spicules of woven bone set in a cellular fibroblastic background with variable number of multinucleated giant cells. This pattern is often associated with secondary hyperparathyroidism related to Chronic renal disease (Renal osteodystrophy).[18]

Treatment and Prognosis:

In primary hyperparathyroidism, the hyperplastic parathyroid tissue or the functional tumor must be removed surgically. Secondary hyperparathyroidism can be controlled by restriction of dietary phosphate, use of phosphate-binding agents, and pharmacologic treatment with an active vitamin D metabolite (e.g., calcitriol).[9]

CHAPTER 18

FIBROUS DYSPLASIA

Fibrous dysplasia (FD) is a benign, non-neoplastic and non-encapsulated fibro-osseous condition involving cranial and extra-cranial bones which show replacement of normal bone by cellular fibrous tissue containing islands of metaplastic bone.[22]

Lichtenstein in 1938 introduced the term Fibrous dysplasia. It is classified by W.H.O. as developmental in origin. Some claim that FD is a dysplastic or hyperplastic process with diffuse margins that blend into adjacent bone. According to some authors, FD is usually caused by mutation in the GNAS1 gene (20q13.2).[18]

FD most frequently occurs in the metaphysial and diaphysial areas of the long bones, the shoulder bones, the bones of the pelvic girdle and those of the jaws and skull. The posterior maxilla is the most common site especially in the area around the first molar. The anterior maxilla is rarely involved. Mandibular lesions are ordinarily found between the mental foramen and angle of the mandible.[85]

In FD, the regular spongiosa is replaced by a fibrous and osseous tissue which is ill suited for expanding and contracting pressure. The cortex becomes narrower due to endosteal bone resorption which can lead to pathological fracture.[10]

Fibrous Dysplasia has been traditionally classified as:[18]

1) Monostotic: Involving only one bone,
2) Polyostotic: Involving more than one bone.

Polyostotic FD is sub-classified as:-

a) Jaffe's type - Many bones are affected and light brown spots over skin i.e. cafe-au- lait spots.
b) Albright syndrome - Several bones are involved with cafe-au-lait spots or lesions in the affected area and along this endocrine dysfunction, like precocious puberty in females.

c) Craniofacial form - Involving the craniofacial complex only.

d) Cherubism

Monostotic Fibrous Dysplasia

This term is applied to those forms of the disease in which only one bone is affected. It occurs in about 70 - 80 % of the cases of FD. It does not manifest extra-skeletal lesions, but may become polyostotic and affect multiple bones. It is less serious than polyostotic form. The clinical term "*leontiasis ossea*" has been applied to cases of Monostotic FD which affects maxilla or facial bones and give the patient a leonine appearance.[9]

Clinical features:

It occurs with equal predilection in males and females with a mild predominance for females. It is more common in children and young adults. Mean age of occurrence being 27-34 years.[85] The first clinical sign of the disease is a painless swelling or bulging of the jaw. The swelling usually involves buccal and labial plate and seldom the lingual plate. When it involves the mandible, it sometimes causes a protuberant excrescence of the inferior border. The overlying mucosa is almost invariably intact over the lesion. Tenderness ultimately develops. There may be some malalignment, tipping or displacement of the teeth due to the progressive expansile nature of the lesion.[10]

Radiographic features:

The roentgenographic appearance of F.D of the jaw is extremely variable. These are 3 basic patterns which may be seen.[18]

In one type, the lesion is generally a rather small unilocular radiolucency or a somewhat larger multilocular radiolucency, due to marked fibrous proliferation and deposition of osteoid which will subsequently calcify. In second type, the pattern is similar except that increased trabeculation renders the lesion more opaque and typically mottled in appearance. Third type is quite opaque, with many delicate trabeculae giving a ground glass or peau d' orange appearance to the lesion. This type is not well circumscribed but blends into the adjacent normal bone.[10]

In all the three types, cortical bone becomes thinned because of the expansile nature of the growth but this bony plate is seldom perforated.[9]

Histopathological features:

The lesion is essentially a fibrous one made up of proliferating fibroblasts in a compact stroma of interlacing collagen fibers.

The trabeculae are thin and located at regular intervals. Irregular trabeculae of bone are scattered through out the lesion, with no definite pattern of arrangement. Characteristically some of these trabeculae are delicate C-shaped or as Chinese character-shaped hook or horse shoe shaped and occasionally may form rings. The trabeculae are usually coarse woven bone but may be lamellar bone. The relationship of osteoblasts and osteoclasts to the trabeculae is similar to that of polyostotic form.[18]

The presence of lamellar bone does not confirm a diagnosis of FD. Other morphological forms of calcification, including small rounded bodies (cementum bodies or globular calcifications) and minute basophilic and laminated calcification may be seen in FD. The histopathology of FD is not pathognomonic and it should be confirmed by correlation of histopathology, radiography and clinical features. Giant cells may also be seen in some cases.[9]

Treatment:

The treatment consists of conservative surgical removal of the lesion. It is estimated that between 25% and 50% of patients will show some regrowth after a conservative surgical procedure. Radiation therapy is contraindicated, as it carries the risk of post irradiation bone sarcoma.

Polyostotic Fibrous Dysplasia (McCUNE ALBRIGHT SYNDROME)

Weil in 1922, recognized the case of polyostotic FD associated with skin lesions and endocrine disturbance. The condition has been specifically described by Albright, from where the apparent syndrome derives its eponym. 'Polyostotic' have been applied to those lesions in which more than one bone is affected.[9]

Clinical features:

It occurs in about 20-30% cases of FD. The disease usually manifests early in life with an evident deformity of long bones, often unilateral in distribution. It has insidious onset. Recurrent bone pain is the most common presenting skeletal symptoms.[64]

Because of the severe bone changes, spontaneous fractures are a common complication of the disease. The structural integrity of the bone is weakened and the weight bearing areas become bowed. The curvature of the femoral neck and proximal shaft of the femur markedly increase causing a *'shepherd crook deformity'*, which is a characteristic sign of the disease. Overgrowth of adjacent soft tissues may be present. Two apparently separate types of polyostotic FD are described as–[18]

Jaffe's type- FD involving a variable number of bones, accompanied by pigmented lesions of the skin or "*cafe-au-lait*" spots of thin light brown color. It is mild and non- progressive form. This type occurs in about 50% of the cases.[97]

Albright's syndrome- FD even more severe, involving nearly all bones in the skeleton accompanied by pigmented lesions of the skin with endocrine disturbances of varying types. Female patients exhibit precocious puberty, sometimes beginning at the age of 2 or 3 years. Vaginal bleeding is a common manifestation.

Oral manifestations:

The oral manifestations of PFD are related to severe disturbance of bony tissue. One third of the polyostotic patients have lesions in the mandible. There may be expansion and deformity of the jaws and the eruption pattern of the teeth is disturbed because of loss of support of the developing teeth. The endocrine disturbance also, may alter the time of eruption of the teeth.

Histological features:

Histological features are similar to that of Monostotic FD. The lesion is composed of fibrillar connective tissue within which numerous trabeculae, woven immature bone, irregular in shape, can be seen.[9]

The osteocytes are quite large and collagen fibers of these trabeculae can often be observed extending into fibrous tissue. Bone formation by stellate osteoblasts can be seen but rows of cuboidal osteoblasts remaining on the surface of the trabeculae (osteoblastic rimming) are absent. These trabeculae typically have wide osteoid seams. Osteoclastic activity may also be seen in some areas.[18]

Laboratory findings:

No consistent and significant changes in serum calcium or phosphorous can be seen, although, serum alkaline phosphatase level is sometimes elevated. Premature secretion of pituitary follicle stimulating hormone is found. There may be an elevated basal metabolic rate.[85]

Treatment:

Mild cases may be treated surgically. Severe forms are treated with X-ray radiation with some success but it is hazardous because of the possibility of development of induced osteosarcomas.[18]

CHAPTER 19

PAGET'S DISEASE

(Paget's disease of bone, osteitis deformans)

Paget's disease is a metabolic disorder affecting the bones. It causes a malfunction in the normal process of bone remodeling. Paget's disease is named after Sir James Paget, an English surgeon who described the clinical course of this disorder and originally named the condition '*osteitis deformans*', as he believed the disease was caused by chronic inflammation.[86]

Paget's disease of bone is characterized by enhanced resorption of bone by giant multinucleated osteoclasts with formation of disorganized woven bone by osteoblasts. This process evolves through various phases of activity, followed by a quiescent stage. Hence, Paget's disease typically consists of the following three phases: (i) Lytic (ii) Mixed lytic and blastic (iii) Sclerotic or burned out.[18]

Clinical features:

The prevalence of Paget's disease increases with age. Paget's disease is recognized most commonly after the age of 50 years and is rarely diagnosed in people younger than 40 years. By the ninth decade of life, prevalence reaches nearly 10% of the peer group. The male to female ratio is approximately 1:1.[87]

A large number of patients in the community are asymptomatic or have mild/unrecognized symptoms. Paget's disease has a predilection for the axial skeleton and may be widespread at the time of diagnosis. The condition commonly affects the pelvis and spine, particularly the lumbar spine with a frequency of 30-75%.[87]

Pain is the most common presenting symptom and may arise from bone affected by pagetic lesions, arthritic or distorted joint architecture, fissure or complete fracture and neurological compression syndromes.[88] The bone pain is perceived as a dull constant aching pain deep below the soft tissues. It may persist or exacerbate during the night. The involved bones become warm to touch because of the increased vascularity.[22]

Other typical findings may include the following: pathologic fractures commonly result from weakened pagetic bone, nonspecific headaches, impaired hearing and tinnitus are common symptoms with skull involvement. The patient's hat size may increase or change due to skeletal deformity and enlargement, especially of the skull bones. Cranial nerve palsies can affect nerves other than the auditory nerve. Change in vision can occur secondary to optic nerve involvement. Back and neck pain are common complaints, as Paget's disease frequently affects the spine, especially the lumbar and sacral regions. Softened bone at the base of the skull may lead to platybasia, the descent of the cranium onto the cervical spine. Progressive pain, paresthesias, limb paresis, gait difficulties (waddling gait) or bowel and bladder incontinence may be caused by compression of the spinal cord or spinal nerve secondary to platybasia or vertebral fractures. Nausea, dizziness, syncope, ataxia, incontinence and dementia can be observed with hydrocephalus, basilar invagination and cerebellar or brainstem compressive syndromes.

Involvement of the facial bones is occasionally seen. It has sometimes been called *leontiasis ossea* (lion-like facies) but because this term is nonspecific, Drury advocated discontinuing its use in referring to this disease.[18]

Oral Manifestations:

Involvement of the jaws in osteitis deformans is a rather common occurrence. There is predilection for the maxilla; the ratio of involvement of maxilla to mandible is approximately 2.3:1. The maxilla exhibits progressive enlargement, the alveolar ridge becomes widened and the palate is flattened. The teeth become loose and migrate, producing spacing in between the teeth. When the mandible is involved, the findings are similar but usually not as severe as in the maxilla. As the disease progresses, the mouth may remain open, exposing the teeth because the lips are too small to cover the enlarged jaw.

Edentulous patients with dentures commonly complain of an inability to wear their appliances because of increasing tightness due to expansion of the jaw. The dentures may to be remade periodically. When the jaws are involved by Paget's disease, there may be involvement of the skull also.[9]

Roentgenographic features:

Paget's disease has sometimes been described as a disorder characterized by an initial phase of deossification and softening followed by a bizarre, dysplastic type of reossification not related to functional requirements, the two processes taking place simultaneously or alternately.[63] These destructive lesions may be multiple and diffuse or isolated. The isolated lesion in the skull, when large, is sometimes referred to as 'osteoporosis circumscripta'. The osteoblastic areas, which appear as opacities in the roentgenogram, tend to be patchy in distribution. This patchiness has been termed a 'cotton-wool' appearance and is especially well demonstrated in the skull and jaws.

Although the disease is usually bilateral, it may show evidence of only unilateral involvement of the jaw, especially early in the course of the disease. The teeth show a rather pronounced hypercementosis, and loss of a well-defined lamina dura around the teeth. Root resorption has been reported in some cases, but this is unusual.[3]

Laboratory findings:

The serum calcium and serum phosphorus levels are usually within normal limits even in cases of advanced osteitis deformans. The serum alkaline phosphatase level may be elevated to over 250 Bodansky units. The serum acid phosphatase level is not increased. Urinary hydroxyproline levels are elevated as they reflect increased osteoclastic activity and bone resorption.[87]

Histologic features:

The initial osteolytic phase is marked by disordered areas of resorption by an increased number of large osteoclasts. These abnormal osteoclasts may contain upto 100 nuclei. The subsequent osteoblastic phase follows with haphazard laying of new bone matrix and formation of woven bone without patterns of stress in between. Repeated episodes of bone removal and formation results in the appearance of many small irregularly shaped bone fragments that appear to be joined in a jigsaw or mosaic pattern with deeply staining hematoxyphilic reversal lines. This pattern is the histologic hallmark of Paget's disease. As the disease progresses, the osteoblastic phase predominates and excessive abnormal bone formation occurs, causing more compact and dense bone. The pagetic bone is coarse and fibrous, with avidity for calcium and phosphorous. Marrow spaces are filled with loose highly vascularized connective tissue. The hypervascular bone combined with cutaneous vasodilation causes an increase in the regional blood flow and accounts for the rise in skin temperature.[9]

The normal trabecular appearance is distorted with a mosaic pattern of irregular cement lines joining areas of lamellar bone. Pagetic bone shows no tendency to form haversian systems. Eventually, the osteoblastic activity diminishes and an osteoporotic or burned-out phase predominates. The new bone is disordered, poorly mineralized, and lacks structural integrity. The proliferation of bone and concomitant hypercementosis sometimes result in obliteration of the periodontal ligament space.[18]

Treatment and Prognosis:

Calcitonin can be used which suppresses bone resorption. Biphosphonates have also been used with some success. Prognosis of the patients with Paget's disease is good if the treatment is administered before major changes in the bones have occurred.[18]

CHAPTER 20

CHERUBISM

(Familial fibrous dysplasia of the jaws, disseminated juvenile fibrous dysplasia, familial multilocular cystic disease of the jaws, familial fibrous swelling of the jaws)

Cherubism is an uncommon, benign fibroosseous lesion which causes a progressive, painless, symmetrical expansion of the jaws. It is primarily found in the mandible. The disease was first described in 1933 by Jones, who called it familial multilocular disease of the jaws. According to the WHO classification, cherubism belongs to a group of non-neoplastic bone lesions affecting only the jaws. It is a rare, benign condition with autosomal dominant inheritance, and it is one of the very few genetically determined osteoclastic lesions in the human body. It appears to have 100 percent penetrance in males and only 50-70% penetrance in females with 2:1 male predominance.[10]

There is great variation in the clinical expression. Although the condition is known to be hereditary, in some cases there has been no detectable family history, and although it usually occurs bilaterally there have also been cases of unilateral involvement, perhaps because of incomplete penetrance or new mutations. Some investigators believe that cherubism arises from the mutation of a nonsex-linked gene responsible for the development of the jaw bones. The specific gene related to cherubism was located on chromosome 4p 16.3, which encodes the SH3 binding protein, SH3 BP2.[4]

Clinical features:

Affected children are normal at birth and are without clinically or radiographically evident disease until 14 months to three years of age. At that time, symmetric enlargement of the jaw begins. Typically, earlier the lesion appears, more rapidly it progresses. The self-limited bone growth usually begins to slow down when the patient reaches five years of age, and stop by the age of 12-15 years. At puberty the lesions begin to regress. Jaw remodeling continues through the third decade of life, at the end of which the clinical abnormality may be subtle. The signs and symptoms depend on the severity of the condition and range from clinically or radiologically undetectable features i.e. mandibular and maxillary overgrowth with respiratory obstruction to impairment of vision and hearing, difficulty in speech and swallowing. Arnott (1978) suggested the following grading system for the lesions of cherubism: Grade I is characterized by involvement of both mandibular ascending rami, Grade II by involvement of both maxillary tuberosities as well as the mandibular ascending rami and Grade III by McCune-Albright syndrome involvement of the whole maxilla and mandible except the coronoid process and condyles.[4]

Another grading system has been proposed by Marck PA (1992) that is – Grade 1 – involvement of both mandibular ascending rami. Grade 2 - involvement of both mandibular ascending rami and both maxillary tuberosities. Grade 3 – massive involvement of the entire maxilla and mandible except the condylar processes. Grade 4 – same as Grade 3 with involvement of the orbits causing orbital compression.[10]

The jaw lesions are usually painless, symmetric and have florid maxillary involvement. The lesions are firm on palpation, nontender, bilaterally symmetrical, most commonly involve the molar to coronoid regions, the condyles always being spared, and are often associated with cervical lymphadenopathy.[80] Enlargement of the cervical lymph nodes contribute to the patient's full-faced appearance and is said to be caused by lymphoid hyperplasia with fibrosis. The lymph nodes become enlarged before the patient reaches six years of age, decrease in size after the age of eight years and are rarely enlarged after the age of 12 years. Intraoral swelling of the alveolar ridges may occur. When the maxillary ridge is involved, the palate assumes a V shape. A rim of sclera may be visible beneath the iris, giving the classic 'eye to heaven' appearance.

In lab investigations for Cherubism, serum calcium and phosphorous levels are within normal limits but alkaline phosphatase levels may be elevated.[18]

Oral Manifestations:

Numerous dental abnormalities, such as agenesis of the second and third molars of the mandible, displacement of the teeth, premature exfoliation of the primary teeth, delayed eruption of the permanent teeth, and transpositions and rotation of the teeth have been reported. In severe cases, tooth resorption may also occur. The deciduous dentition may be shed prematurely, beginning as early as three years of age. The permanent dentition is often defective, with absence of numerous teeth and displacement and lack of eruption of those present. The oral mucosa is usually intact and of normal color. Although cherubism was initially described as a familial disease affecting the jaws, cases without any apparent hereditary origin have been reported. In a few cases, cherubism has been described as being connected with other diseases and conditions such as **Noonan's syndrome,** a lesion in the humerus, gingival fibromatosis, psychomotor retardation, orbital involvement and obstructive sleep apnea. The association between these two rare inherited diseases suggests that these are independent diseases that may be transmitted by genes closely linked on the same chromosome.[9]

Roentgenographic Features:

Radiographically, cherubism is characterized by bilateral multilocular, radiolucent, cystic expansion of the jaws. Early lesions occur in the posterior body of the mandible and the ascending rami. Maxillary lesions may occur at the same time but escape early radiographic detection because of overlap of the sinus and nasal cavities. Displacement of the inferior alveolar canal has been reported. The presence of numerous unerupted teeth and the destruction of the alveolar bone may displace the teeth, producing a radiographic appearance referred to as 'floating tooth syndrome'. With adulthood, the cystic areas in the jaws become re-ossified, which results in irregular patchy sclerosis. There is a classic (but nonspecific) ground glass appearance because of the small, tightly compressed trabecular pattern.[10]

Histologic Features:

Histologic examination of the lesions usually reveals numerous multinucleated giant cells. These multinucleated cells show strong positivity for tartarate resistant acid phosphatase, which is characteristic of osteoclasts. The collagenous stroma, which contains a large number of spindle-shaped fibroblasts, is considered unique because of its water-logged, granular nature. Numerous small vessels are present, and the capillaries exhibit large endothelial cells and perivascular cuffing. The eosinophilic cuffing appears to be specific to cherubism. However, these deposits are not present in many cases, and their absence does not exclude the diagnosis of cherubism. Older, resolving lesions of cherubism show an increase in fibrous tissue, a decrease in the number of giant cells and formation of new bone. The microscopic findings seldom permit a specific diagnosis of cherubism in the absence of clinical and radiological information.[22]

Treatment:

Surgery to correct the jaw deformities of cherubism is rarely indicated. If necessary, surgery is usually undertaken after puberty, when the remission phase of the lesions has been reached, unless esthetic considerations or severe functional problems justify earlier treatment. Although exacerbation has sometimes been reported after surgery, it is believed that surgery ultimately accelerates the involution process.[9]

CHAPTER 21

GIANT CELL FIBROMA

Giant cell fibroma (GCF) is a benign non-neoplastic lesion first described by Weathers and Callihan (1974). The GCF is a fibrous tumor with distinctive clinicopathologic features. Unlike the traumatic fibroma, it does not appear to be associated with chronic irritation. The giant cell fibroma represents approximately 2% to 5% of all oral fibrous proliferations submitted for biopsy.[90]

Clinical features:

Giant cell fibroma occurs in the first three decades of life and predominates in females. The GCF is typically an asymptomatic sessile or pedunculated nodule, usually less than 1 cm in size. The surface of the mass often appears papillary; therefore the lesion may be clinically mistaken for a papilloma. Approximately 50% of all the cases occur on the gingiva. The mandibular gingiva is affected twice as often as the maxillary gingiva. The tongue and palate are also common sites.[90]

Histologic Features:

Microscopically, a giant cell fibroma is an unencapsulated mass of loose fibrous connective tissue. The connective tissue contains numerous characteristic large, plump, spindle-shaped and stellate fibroblasts, some of which are multinucleated. These cells are easily observed in the peripheral areas of the lesion, whereas the more central area, contain typical fusiform fibroblasts. The surface epithelium is corrugated and atrophic; in contrast to an irritation fibroma, a giant cell fibroma has a thin, elongated rete ridges.

The origin of stellate and multinucleate cells is not well known. Few studies showed positive immunostaining for vimentin. This suggests that the stellate and multinucleate cells of GCF have a fibroblast phenotype.[18]

Treatment and Prognosis:

Conservative excisional biopsy is curative, and its findings are diagnostic. Recurrence is rare.

NODULAR FASCIITIS

Nodular fasciitis, also known as *pseudosarcomatous fasciitis,* is a well-recognized entity representing a fibrous connective tissue growth. A closely related lesion known as *proliferative myositis* occurs in muscle. The cause of this proliferation is unknown. Trauma is believed to be important in many cases because of the location of lesions over bony prominences, such as the angle of the mandible and the zygoma. Although traditionally considered a reactive condition, recent molecular evidence suggests that the cells in nodular fasciitis are clonal, thus supporting the concept that the lesion is a benign neoplasm.[18]

Clinical features:

The lesion typically presents as a firm mass in the dermis or the submucosa and exhibits such rapid growth clinically that malignancy may be suspected. Pain or tenderness often accompanies the process. There is no gender predilection, and young adults and adults are usually affected. The trunk and extremities are the areas most commonly involved, with about 10% of cases appearing in the head and neck, usually in the skin of the face and the parotid sheath. All of these lesions are benign and if left untreated ultimately regress on their own. Local recurrence occurs in only 2% of cases.[18]

Histopathology:

Encapsulation is lacking, and poor circumscription often is a notable feature, most strikingly in the form of tongue-like projection into the adjacent fat. The lesions are composed of a rather confused admixture of proliferating fibroblasts and capillaries.[91]

A nodular growth contains plump fibroblasts with vesicular nuclei in a haphazard to storiform arrangement. Myxoid areas are often found. Multinucleated giant cells are occasionally present and may originate from adjacent muscle or from fusion of macrophages. They have dull, amphophilic cytoplasm and three to six oval or rounded nuclei. Mitotic figures may be frequent but are morphologically normal in appearance. Inflammatory cells and extravasated red blood cells are also microscopic features of nodular fasciitis.

Proliferative myositis, an analogous lesion occurring within muscle, is a reactive lesion that usually occurs in the trunk and rarely in the head and the neck (sternocleidomastoid muscle). It parallels the clinical course of nodular fasciitis, although it appears in an older age-group.[18]

Differential Diagnosis:

Diagnostic problems relative to nodular fasciitis occur because many of its microscopic features are shared by other fibrous proliferations, such as fibromatosis, fibrous histiocytoma, and fibrosarcoma.

Fibromatosis is more infiltrative than nodular fasciitis and may exhibit a fasicular growth pattern. It also produces more collagen, is generally less cellular, and has fewer mitotic figures. Fibrous histiocytoma is more cellular with a storiform pattern, and it may not be as well circumscribed as nodular fasciitis. Fibrosarcoma is infiltrative and exhibits a Herringbone pattern. Also, nuclei are pleomorphic and hyperchromatic, and mitoses are more abundant and atypical.

By immunohistochemistry, the cells of nodular fasciitis express smooth muscle actin but not desmin. Some have described variable staining with the CD68 marker KPI.[9]

Treatment:

Conservative surgical excision is the treatment of choice for nodular fasciitis. Recurrences are rarely encountered.

CHAPTER 22

EPULIS FISSURATUM

(Inflammatory Fibrous Hyperplasia; Denture Injury Tumor; Denture Epulis)

The epulis fissuratum is a tumorlike hyperplasia of fibrous connective tissue that develops in association with the flange of an ill-fitting complete or partial denture. Although the simple term epulis sometimes is used synonymously for epulis fissuratum, epulis is actually a generic term that can be applied to any tumor of the gingiva or alveolar mucosa. Therefore, some authors prefer to call these lesions inflammatory fibrous hyperplasia.[9]

Clinical Features:

The epulis fissuratum typically appears as a single or multiple fold or folds of hyperplastic tissue in the alveolar vestibule. Most often, there are two folds of tissue, and the flange of the associated denture fits conveniently into the fissure between the folds. The redundant tissue is usually firm and fibrous, although some lesions appear erythematous and ulcerated similar to the appearance of a pyogenic granuloma. Occasional examples of epulis fissuratum demonstrate surface areas of inflammatory papillary hyperplasia. The size of the lesion can vary from localized hyperplasias less than 1 cm in size to massive lesions that involve most of the length of the vestibule. The epulis fissuratum usually develops on the facial aspect of the alveolar ridge, although occasional lesions are seen lingual to the mandibular alveolar ridge.

The epulis fissuratum most often occurs in middle aged and older adults. It may occur on either the maxilla or mandible. The anterior portion of the jaws is affected much more often than the posterior areas. There is a pronounced female predilection; most studies show that two thirds to three fourths of all cases submitted for biopsy occur in women.[18]

Another similar but less common fibrous hyperplasia, often called a fibroepithelial polyp or leaflike denture fibroma, occurs on the hard palate beneath a maxillary denture. This characteristic lesion is a flattened pink mass that is attached to the palate by a narrow stalk. Usually, the flattened mass is closely applied to the palate and sits in a slightly cupped out depression. However, it is easily lifted up with a probe, which demonstrates its pedunculated nature. The edge of the lesion often is serrated and resembles a leaf.[18]

Histopathologic features:

Microscopic examination of the epulis fissuratum reveals hyperplasia of the fibrous connective tissue. Often multiple folds and grooves occur where the denture impinges on the tissue. The overlying epithelium is frequently hyperparakeratotic with irregular hyperplasia of the rete ridges. In some instances, the epithelium shows inflammatory papillary hyperplasia or pseudoepitheliomatous (pseudocarcinomatous) hyperplasia. Focal areas of ulceration are not unusual, especially at the base of the grooves between the folds. A variable chronic inflammatory infiltrate is present; sometimes, it may include eosinophils or show lymphoid follicles. If minor salivary glands are included in the specimen, they usually show chronic sialadenitis.[9]

Surface epithelium shows *mucopolysaccharide keratin dystrophy,* also referred to as 'plasma pooling', first described by Toto. This mucopolysaccharide keratin dystrophy consists histologically of homogeneous, eosinophilic pools of material in the superficial spinous layer of epithelium, where it appears to have replaced individual cells.[18]

In rare instances, the formation of osteoid or chondroid is observed. This as osseous and chondromatous metaplasia, is a reactive phenomenon caused by chronic irritation by the ill-fitting denture. The denture-related fibroepithelial polyp has a core of dense fibrous connective tissue covered by hyperplastic stratified squamous epithelium.[9]

Treatment and Prognosis:

Lesion has to be surgically excised. New dentures have to be constructed.

CHAPTER 23

TRAUMATIC GRANULOMA

(Eosinophilic ulceration, Traumatic ulcerative granuloma with stromal eosinophilia [TUGSE])

Acute or chronic trauma to the oral mucosa may result in surface ulcerations. The ulcerations may remain for extended periods of time, but most usually heal within days. These exhibits a deep pseudoinvasive inflammatory reaction and is typically slow to resolve.

In addition, similar sublingual ulcerations may occur in infants as a result of chronic mucosal trauma from adjacent anterior primary teeth, often associated with nursing. These distinctive ulcerations of infancy have been termed Riga Fede disease and are a variation of the traumatic eosinophilic ulceration.

In most cases of traumatic ulceration, there is an adjacent source of irritation, although this is not present invariably. The clinical presentation often suggests the cause, but many cases resemble early ulcerative squamous cell carcinoma; biopsy is performed to rule out that possibility.[93]

Clinical features:

Traumatic granuloma (TG) is commonly observed in all age groups, with a significant male preponderance. They are usually seen in the anteroventral and dorsal surfaces of the tongue. Lesions may also be observed in other sites such as the gingiva, the palate and the mucobuccal fold.

Traumatic granuloma is a chronic, benign, self-limiting lesion of the oral mucosa, manifesting as an ulcer with elevated margins.[53] The ulcerations usually persist up to a week or even up to eight months. They resemble the simple traumatic ulcerations, appearing as area of erythema surrounding a central removable yellow fibropurulent membrane. Further, rolled borders of hyperorthokeratosis may develop immediately adjacent to the area of ulceration. The proliferation of the underlying granulation tissue can lead to a raised lesion resembling pyogenic granuloma.[93]

Histological features:

Simple traumatic ulcerations are covered by a fibrinopurulent membrane that consists of fibrin intermixed with neutrophils. The membrane is of variable thickness. The adjacent surface epithelium may be normal or may demonstrate slight hyperplasia with or without hyperkeratosis.

Microscopically, TG is characterized by a dense polymorphic inflammatory infiltrate extending into the underlying muscle. The dominant cell types in the inflammatory infiltrate are small lymphocytes, with abundant eosinophils.

Mucosal degeneration is characteristic and may be attributed to proliferation of cytotoxic T cells or toxic products released by degranulating eosinophils. This degenerated mucosa permits the ingress of microorganisms, toxins, and foreign proteins into the connective tissue. In predisposed persons, these substances induce a severe inflammatory response resulting from an exaggerated mast cell-eosinophil reaction similar to that noticed in the pathogenesis of bronchial asthma.

The presence of large, atypical mononuclear cells is another microscopic feature of TG present in most cases. The origin of these large cells has been a matter of debate. Some scientists believe them to be of macrophage origin and some say that they represent myofibroblasts.[94]

Treatment and Prognosis:

For traumatic ulcerations that have an obvious source of injury, the irritating cause should be removed. If the cause is not obvious or if a patient does not respond to therapy, biopsy is indicated. Rapid healing after a biopsy is typical even with large eosinophilic ulcerations. Recurrence is not expected.[9]

CHAPTER 24

OSTEOMALACIA

A deficiency of vitamin D function in *adults* impairs or blocks the normal mineralization of osteoid laid down in the remodelling of bone, producing *osteomalacia*. In *growing children*, not only is there inadequate mineralization of osteiod, but also there is inadequate provisional mineralization of epiphyseal cartilage, inducing *rickets*. Osteomalacia is characterized by incomplete mineralization of normal osteoid tissue following closure of the growth plates.[8]

Clinical features:

Rickets and osteomalacia are different manifestations of the same underlying pathologic process, depending on whether the patient is a child or an adult, respectively. Clinically, osteomalacia is subtler than rickets, particularly in mild or moderate disease. Mildly affected patients may present with nonspecific bone pain and tenderness and possibly hypotonia. Severely affected patients may have difficulty ambulating and may walk with a waddling gait. Milkman syndrome is a condition in which the patient experiences multiple insufficiency fractures that are often bilateral and symmetric.[2]

Histological features:

Osteomalacia is marked by inadequate mineralization and hence an excess of unmineralized osteoid, this zone is called as Looser's zones. The basic defect in bone and bone growth is a failure of mineralization. The so-called diagnostic feature histologically is the osteoid seam, a layer of unmineralized bone surrounding mineralized bone. There is an attempt at bone remodeling with inadequate calcification of bone matrix. The cortical bone is thin and osteoid borders are found on the trabeculae.[18]

Treatment:

Treatment involves the administration, in appropriate amounts and combinations, of vitamin D, calcium, phosphate, and alkalinizing solutions. Orthopaedic measures may be required to correct deformities that cannot be expected to improve with growth.[18]

ANEURYSMAL BONE CYST

The aneurysmal bone cyst (ABC) is an uncommon lesion which has been found in most bones of the skeleton.[95] Jaffe and Lichtenstein were the first to recognize ABC as an intraosseous, osteolytic lesion chiefly affecting the metaphyseal region of long bones and vertebrae.[96] The term 'aneurysmal bone cyst' was suggested by Jaffe and Lichenstein (1942),[95] the word "aneurysmal" to emphasize the "blown-out," distended contour of the affected bone, and the words "bone cyst" to underscore that when the lesion is entered through a thin shell of bone, it appears largely as a blood-filled cavity.[97]

According to Clough and Price (1968) the majority of lesions occur in long bones and in the spine. Bernier and Bhaskar (1958) described the first case of ABC involving the craniofacial skeleton.[95] Only 1.9% of all ABCs occur in the jaws, representing 1.5% of all nonodontogenic cysts.[96]

The **World Health Organization** defines aneurysmal bone cyst (ABC) as "*a benign tumour-like lesion with an expanding osteolytic lesion consisting of blood-filled spaces of variable size separated by connective tissue septa containing trabeculae or osteoid tissue and osteoclast giant cells*". Although benign, ABC can be a rapidly growing and destructive bone lesion. The expansile nature of this lesion can cause pain, swelling, deformity, perforation or disruption of cortical plates, neurological symptoms (depending on its location) and pathologic fracture.[96]

Pathogenesis:

The pathogenesis of the aneurysmal bone cyst is controversial and number of theories has been proposed. The original cases reported by Jaffe and

Lichtenstein (1942) were in the long bones and showed eccentric bone expansion indicating a juxtacortical or subperiosteal lesion.[95]

Subsequently, it has become apparent that the aneurysmal bone cyst may have a juxtacortical or intramedullary location. Kransdorf and Sweet (1995) have led to the concept of aneurysmal bone cyst being the end result of a common pathophysiological process with a variety of causes. Juxta-cortical lesions that are found in a subperiosteal location are thought to be primarily of traumatic origin, whereas intramedullary lesions reflect secondary change within pre-existing lesions. Juxtacortical lesions have not been reported in the head and neck and although trauma has been postulated, there is little evidence to support this as a cause of jaw lesions. Kransdorf and Sweet (1995) suggested that the cysts may result from a vascular disturbance in the form of sudden venous occlusion or the development of an arteriovenous shunt. This would usually occur in more vascular, newly formed parts of the immature skeleton and in a preexisting lesion.[95]

The concept of aneurysmal bone cyst as a secondary phenomenon occurring in a pre-existing lesion has been validated by multiple investigators; in approximately one third (29-35%) of cases, the pre-existing lesion can be identified. The most common of these is giant cell tumor, which accounts for 19-39% of those cases in which the preceding lesion is found. Other common precursor lesions include osteoblastoma, angioma, and chondroblastoma. Less common lesions include fibrous dysplasia, fibroxanthoma (nonossifying fibroma), chondromyxoid fibroma, solitary bone cyst, fibrous histiocytoma, eosinophilic granuloma, radiation osteitis, osteosarcoma, trauma (including fracture), fibrosarcoma, and even metastatic carcinoma.

Other investigators have proposed two forms of aneurysmal bone cyst, those in which the lesion is secondary to an identifiable precursor, and a "primary aneurysmal bone cyst" in which no pre-existing lesion is identified.

Much of the controversy surrounding this lesion may be the result of a change in how the lesion was defined by Lichenstein in 1953, when intramedullary lesions were added to previously described juxtracortical (superficial) lesion.[97]

Struthers and Shear (1984) suggested that the initiating change in the primary lesion appeared to be the microcyst. They pointed out that the formation of microcysts in fibrous dysplasia had been described by Geschickter and Copeland (1949), Jaffe (1953) and Fisher (1976). The central giant cell granuloma has a propensity to form micro cysts because of its loose, oedematous, fibrillar connective tissue stroma in which lie many thin-walled blood vessels and extravasated erythrocytes. Microcyst formation is facilitated by localised areas of necrosis in the stroma brought about by stagnation and ischaemia. The resulting micro cysts are lined by stromal connective tissue and in giant cell lesions multinucleate giant cells may form part of their margins. They enlarge by further stromal breakdown and coalesce with each other. Loss of stromal support leads to dilatation and rupture of the thin-walled vessels and haemorrhage into the stroma and the microcysts. An association of dilated blood vessels and microcysts is frequently observed.[95]

Once a vascular connection is established between a larger vessel and a microcyst, haemodynamic pressure participates in its enlargement and little supportive resistance is offered if the surrounding stroma is loose and oedematous. The spaces now assume the dimensions of macrocysts which are surrounded by a layer of compressed stroma and these multiple expanding blood-filled cysts produce a pressure resorption of bone. Endosteal resorption of the cortical plates occurs ultimately and once these are breached a 'blowout' of the lesion, covered with periosteum, occurs. A layer of periosteal new bone may be deposited to form a thin shell covering the aneurysmal bone cyst.[95]

Struthers and Shear (1984) were of the opinion that a malignant lesion was less likely to produce the classic clinicopathological features of an aneurysmal bone cyst because of its tendency to break out of bone. The rare development of aneurysmal bone cyst in malignant lesions probably explains the so-called malignant form of the cyst occasionally reported in the literature (Levy et at., 1975).[95]

To conclude this discussion of the possible pathogenesis of the aneurysmal bone cyst, it should be stated that there are a number of authorities who dispute the theory that the cyst is a secondary phenomenon.[95]

Chromosomal translocation t(16;17) (q22;p13) can be seen as a recurring abnormality in aneurysmal bone cyst indicating that some of the lesions are neoplastic. Nonrandom rearrangements of chromosomes bands 16q22 and 17p13 are observed in solid variant of ABC and extraosseous ABC suggesting that the entire spectrum of ABCs probably shares a common pathogenesis.[98]

Clinical Features:

The aneurysmal bone cyst is generally a lesion of young persons, predominantly occurring under the age of 20 years. The lesion can be encountered in adults as well.[97] ABCs are found more frequently in the mandible than the maxilla (3:1) with preponderance for the body, ramus and angle of the mandible. Involvement of other bones of the face such as zygoma and zygomatic arch has also been reported.[96]

There is no significant predilection for either gender.[18] However recent studies have indicated an increased incidence in females.[97] The lesions are usually tender or painful, particularly upon motion, and this soreness may limit movement of the affected bone. Swelling over the area of bone involvement is also common.[97]

Occasionally, there is a history of recent displacement of teeth, which remain vital. When the lesion perforates the cortex and is covered by periosteum or only a thin shell of bone, it may exhibit springiness or egg shell crackling, but is not pulsatile. Bruits are not heard. Patient may complain of some degree trismus or temporo mandibular joint pain. This can be attributed to the physical impringement of the lesion on the joint capsule.[95]

Gross findings at the time of operation are characteristic. Upon entering the lesion, excessive bleeding is encountered, the blood 'welling up' from the tissue. The tissue has been described as resembling a blood-soaked sponge with large pores representing the cavernous spaces of the lesion. In manometric studies by Biesecker and his associates, some of the cysts had elevated vascular pressures as high as arteriolar levels. According to Shafer a history of traumatic injury preceding development of the lesion may often be obtained.[18]

The cyst contains variable amount of soft tissue consisting of friable vascular tissue which subdivides the cavity into a number of blood filled locules. Part of the lesion may contain areas of more solid tissue. These may represent either areas of repair or remnants of a pre-existing lesion. No direct communication with any vessels can be demonstrated at operation.[95]

Histological features:

Dabska M, Buraczewski J (1968) observed that the excised part of the bone looked like an inflated balloon with raised periosteum. Immediately underneath the periosteum a thin osseous shell was present and covered the entire tumor. Under the shell the bone was completely destroyed and replaced by a labyrinth of rounded cavities of various sizes filled with large quantities of liquid blood.[99]

On section aneurysmal bone cyst presents the appearance of a cavernous vascular tumor. In long bones the eccentric localization is evident. The cavities are surrounded by whitish-gray or brownish elastic fibrous tissue. The diameter of the cavities is from a few mm to 1 or 2 cm. The inner surfaces are smooth and glossy. The cavities are intercommunicating and do not contain clots. In some cases structural differences may appear. Some tumors have a strikingly cystic character with multiple small cysts divided by scanty fibrous connective tissue. On section some tumors resemble a sponge, while others are more fibrous with fewer cavities and look like Swiss cheese. In the fibrous tissue dividing the cavities some osseous elements may be seen even with the naked eye.[99]

Microscopic features may differ in detail from case to case. In the resected tumor the most striking picture is the presence of multiple large and small cavities of various sizes, some swollen and filled with blood, others empty with loose walls or filled with packed proteinaceous material. No tumor has endothelial lining or smooth muscle tissue in the walls of dilated muscular spaces. However, in some tumors many bulging vessels are present-mostly capillaries and give the impression of being under blood pressure.[99]

These vessels and vascular spaces are supported by connective tissue with filamentous trabeculae of newly formed bone. Around the spaces varying numbers of multinuclear giant tells are present. Sometimes they cause the diagnostic error of giant cell tumor. It should be remembered that giant cell tumors (unless irradiated) do not produce osteoid. The presence of osteoid tissue and of bony trabeculae may be taken as evidence against a diagnosis of osteoclastoma. Moreover, the affected bone area, which is composed mostly of blood-filled cavities, is covered by periosteum and outlined by a thin subperiosteal bone shell. The latter feature, although not exclusive to aneurysmal bone cyst, is a constant finding.[99]

In some of the solid areas, sheets of vascular tissue, containing large numbers of multinucleate giant cells, fibroblast, hemorrhage and hemosiderin, look very much like giant cell granuloma of the jaws. Other solid areas may have the appearance of fibrous dysplasia, ossifying fibroma and possibly other jaw tumors. This gives evidence to the view that the aneurysmal bone cyst may represent secondary changes in pre-existing lesion.[95]

According to Clough and Price (1968) there are no cellular features suggestive of malignant neoplasia unless, of course, the cyst has developed in a malignant tumor. Liu et al. (2003) undertook a comparison of the histopathology of giant cell lesions of the jaws and concluded that aneurysmal bone cyst is primarily a giant cell lesion and is related to giant cell granuloma of the jaws.[95]

Radiological features:

The lesion has a characteristic 'ballooning' growth pattern which results in a radiolucent area with elevation of the periosteum to produce an ovoid or fusiform expansion of the bone with the typical 'blown-out' cortical expansion. CT scan reveals a thin uninterrupted cortex.

Lesions are usually unilocular but longer standing lesions may show a 'soap-bubble' appearance and may become progressively calcified. Teeth may be displaced and root resorption may be present. Radiological differentiation from other expansile jaw lesions may be difficult.[95]

Treatment:

The mainstay of treatment is surgery. The majority of patients undergo curettage and bone graft and/or cementation.

CHAPTER 25

CALCIFYING ODONTOGENIC CYST

(Calcifying Cystic Odontogenic Tumor)

The term calcifying odontogenic cyst (COC) was first introduced by Gorlin and his colleagues in 1962. The COC is a developmental odontogenic cyst with diverse origin as either a cyst or a neoplasm.[100]

Calcifying odontogenic cyst was earlier thought to be an oral presentation of cutaneous calcifying epithelioma of Malherbe (1982). It was also termed as '*keratinizing cyst*' and referred as a cyst by Chen & Miller. Gold found keratinization as a prominent feature and therefore renamed the lesion as '*keratinizing and calcifying odontogenic cyst*' (KCOC). Because of the varied histopathologic characteristics, various terminologies have been proposed which includes '*calcifying ghost cell odontogenic tumor*'(CGCOT) proposed by Fejerskov & Krogh in 1972 and '*cystic calcifying odontogenic tumor*' proposed by Freedman et al. (CCOT) in 1975.[101]

Over the years since its first description, it has become clear that the calcifying odontogenic cyst (COC) has a number of variants, including features of a benign odontogenic tumor. It was classified as such, with SNOMED code 9301/0, in the World Health Organization's (WHO) publication *Histological Typing of Odontogenic Tumors* (Kramer *et al.,* 1992). The studies of Praetorius *et al.* (1981) led them to conclude that what had previously been regarded as a calcifying odontogenic cyst actually comprised two entities: a cyst and a neoplasm. In the latest WHO publication on odontogenic tumors (Praetorius and Ledesma-Montes, 2005) it was classified as a benign odontogenic tumor and was renamed '*calcifying cystic odontogenic tumor*' (CCOT).[95]

Suggested classification of the odontogenic ghost cell lesions[95]-

(From *Praetorius, 2006*, personal communication)

Group 1

'Simple' cysts

Calcifying odontogenic cyst (COC)

Group 2

Cysts associated with odontogenic hamartomas or benign neoplasms: calcifying cystic odontogenic tumors (CCOT). The following combinations have been published:

CCOT associated with an odontome

CCOT associated with adenomatoid odontogenic tumor CCOT associated with ameloblastoma

CCOT associated with ameloblastic fibroma

CCOT associated with ameloblastic fibro-odontoma CCOT associated with odonto-ameloblastoma

CCOT associated with odontogenic myxofibroma

Group 3

Solid benign odontogenic neoplasms with similar cell morphology to that in the COC, and with dentinoid formation

Dentinogenic ghost cell tumor

Group 4

Malignant odontogenic neoplasms with features similar to those of the dentinogenic ghost cell tumor

Ghost cell odontogenic carcinoma

Pathogenesis:

The pathogenesis is considerably complicated by the fact that the epithelial lining of a calcifying odontogenic cyst appears to have the ability to induce the formation of dental tissues in the adjacent connective tissue wall; and that other odontogenic tumors such as the ameloblastoma, the odontoameloblastoma, the ameloblastic fibroma and the ameloblastic fibro-odontome may sometimes be associated with it (Praetorius, 1975; Hirshberg *et at.,* 1994; Aithal *et at.,* 2003; Lin *et at.,* 2004; Iida *et at.,* 2004).[95]

Takeda et al. (1990) were convinced that the cysts arose *de novo,* as were Praetorius et al. (1981), who concluded from their study that substantial evidence existed that the tumor developed from the wall of the cyst. They suggested that the calcifying odontogenic cyst was a unicystic process that developed from reduced enamel epithelium or remnants of odontogenic epithelium in the follicle, gingival tissue or bone. Dentinoid alone or an odontome may be found in the cyst wall, induced by the lining epithelium. Praetorius believes that the dentinogenic ghost cell tumor is a neoplasm *de novo,* but the COC plus benign neoplasm or hamartoma is a cyst from the beginning.[95]

Clinical features:

The terms used for the solid neoplastic variant of COC were '*dentinogenic ghost cell tumor*' (DGCT) by Praetorius et al., '*epithelial odontogenic ghost cell tumor*' (EOGCT) by Ellis & Shmookler in 1986, '*odontogenic ghost cell tumor*' (OGCT) proposed by Colmenero et al. in 1990 and '*odontogenic ghost cell ameloblastoma*' by Shear in 1994. The lesion accounts for 1% of all odontogenic jaw cysts. The cystic or non neoplastic variant of COC is found to occur in 80-98%, of cases and associated with odontoma in 24% of cases. The solid or neoplastic variant of COC accounted to about 11.5% of cases. The COC are usually intraosseous (70% of the cases) with extraosseous presentation accounting for 16-22% mostly seen in individuals above the age of 50 years.[101]

The age ranges from 1 year to 82 years with peak in the 2nd decade. In their study Praetorius et al. (1981) and Buchner (1991), have drawn attention to bimodal age distribution with peaks in the second and sixth decades.[95]

The lesion has no sex predilection and is equally distributed between maxilla and mandible. COC are common anterior to the first molar region in which 75% of cases are in the incisor canine region or intercanine region usually crossing the midline of the mandible, which is a rare feature in the maxilla.[101]

Swelling is the most frequent complaint and has occurred in about half of the reported cases. Only rarely has there been pain. Intra-osseous lesions may produce a hard bony expansion and may be fairly extensive. Lingual expansion may sometimes be observed. Occasionally, the calcifying odontogenic cyst may perforate the cortical plate and extend into the soft tissues. In a few cases, displacement of the teeth has been described. Extra-osseous lesions tend to be pink to red, circumscribed elevated masses measuring up to 4cm in diameter.[95]

Radiological features:

The COC that occurs as an intra-osseous lesion appears as an essentially radiolucent area. Some have a regular outline with well-demarcated margins. Others may be quite irregular with poorly defined margins. They are usually unilocular but a few are multilocular. Irregular calcified bodies of varying size and opacity may be seen in the radiolucent area. Denser opacities are likely to be present if the cyst is associated with a complex odontome. Some cases are associated with an unerupted tooth. Displacement of teeth and resorption of the roots of adjacent teeth are frequent findings. Local expansion sometimes occurs and perforation of the cortical plate, when present, may be radiologically demonstrable. The extra-osseous lesions show localized superficial bone resorption, or saucer-shaped radiolucencies and sometimes displacement of adjacent teeth.[95]

Histological features:

The epithelial lining has characteristic odontogenic features with a prominent basal layer consisting of palisaded columnar or cuboidal cells and hyperchromatic nuclei which are polarized away from the basement membrane. The epithelium may be regular 6-8 cells thick over part of its length and be continuous with parts that may be very thin and others that are considerably thickened. Budding from the basal layer into the adjacent connective tissue and epithelial proliferations into the lumen are frequently seen.

The most remarkable feature of the COC is the presence of ghost cells. The ghost cells are found in groups, particularly in the thicker areas of the epithelial lining. The spinous cells in such situations may be widely separated by intercellular oedema and the epithelium around the ghost cells is often convoluted.

The ghost cells are enlarged, ballooned, and ovoid or elongated ellip-toid epithelial cells. They are eosinophillic and although the cell outlines are usually well-defined, they may sometimes be blurred so that groups of them appear fused. A few ghost cells may contain nuclear remnants but these are in various stages of degeneration and in the majority all traces of chromatin have disappeared leaving only a faint outline of the original nucleus. The ghost cells represent an abnormal type of keratinization and have an affinity for calcification. Ghost cells may represent the products of coagulative necrosis of odontogenic epithelium. Sapp and Gardner (1977) found that calcification may occur in some of the ghost cells, ultra structural studies have shown to represent dystrophic calcification.

The ghost cells may be in contact with the connective tissue wall of the cyst where they may then evoke a foreign body reaction with the formation of multinucleate giant cells. In the fibrous wall there are usually strands and islands of odontogenic epithelium, either in direct contact with the epithelium or separately in the connective tissue. An atubular dentinoid is often found in the wall close to the epithelial lining and often in relation to the epithelial proliferations. It is found particularly in contact with masses of ghost cells.[95]

Treatment:

The COC is treated by surgical enucleation unless it is associated with another odontogenic tumor, in which case wider excision may be required. [95]

CHAPTER 26

SOLITARY BONE CYST

(Traumatic bone cyst, Simple bone cyst, Hemorrhagic bone cyst, Extravasation cyst, Unicameral bone cyst, Idiopathic bone cyst)

A solitary bone cyst is an anatomic indentation of the posterior lingual mandible that appears to resemble a cyst on radiographic examination. This depression of the mandible is believed to be developmental in origin. It is an unusual benign, empty or fluid filled cavity within bone that is devoid of epithelial lining.[22]

Clinical features:

The solitary bone cyst is not a common lesion. This cystic lesion is usually asymptomatic and is discovered during routine radiographic examination. In some cases, enlargement of the mandible, most frequently buccal and labial, can be seen.[18]

The simple bone cyst occurs in young individuals. The patients ranged in age from 25 to 35 years. Killey, Kay and Seward recorded a peak frequency in the second decade. Male to female ratio is 1.6:1 and majority of lesions occur in mandible. Almost all the maxillary cases involve the anterior regions and the majority of the mandibular cases have been reported in the body and symphyseal area. In some cases, enlargement of the mandible has been observed.[95]

The pulps of the teeth in the involved area are vital and does not show root resorption. When the cavity is opened surgically, it is found to contain either a small amount of straw colored fluid, shreds of necrotic clot, fragments of fibrous connective tissue or nothing.[9]

Histological features:

The simple bone cyst consists of a thin loose vascular fibrous tissue membrane of variable thickness with no epithelial lining or demonstrates a thickened myxofibromatous proliferation that is often intermixed with trabeculae of cellular and reactive bone. Haemorrhage and haemosiderin pigment are usually present and scattered small multinucleated giant cells are often found. Some cyst walls, possibly cases of longer standing, are more densely fibrous.

The adjacent bone, when included in the specimen, shows osteoclastic resorption (howship's lacunae) on its inner surface. Beasley (1976) described areas of hemorrhage associated with necrotic tissue or tissue showing myxoid degeneration. These occurred in cavities adjacent to areas of bone resorption. Thrombi were not observed in any of the specimens which he examined. Cases associated with florid osseous dysplasia or cemento-osseous dysplasias have been reported.[95]

Treatment:

Simple surgical exploration to establish the diagnosis is usually sufficient therapy for solitary bone cyst of jaws. After surgical exploration with or without curettage of the bony walls, obliteration of the defect by new bone formation is generally rapid. Recurrence or persistence of the lesion is most unusual. The prognosis is, however, excellent.[18]

CHAPTER 27

OSTEOID OSTEOMA

Osteoid osteoma is a benign, solitary, painful circumscribed osteoblastic bone tumor of spongy bone. It was first identified as a clinical entity by Jaffe in 1935. It has been shown that the tumor nidus in osteoid osteomas contains a concentration of peripheral nerves not seen in other fibro-osseous neoplasms. The size of osteoid osteoma is less than 2 cms. Osteoid osteoma and osteoblastoma are closely related benign bone tumors, with osteoid osteoma being under 2 cms and osteoblastoma being larger than 2 cms.

Clinical features:

Osteoid osteoma usually occurs in the second and third decades of life. Men are affected more frequently than women having male to female ratio of at least 2:1. Osteoid osteomas occur most often in the femur, tibia and phalanges. They are very rare in the jaws but if occur, there is mandibular predominance. The body of mandible is affected in most of the cases. They can be classified as cortical, cancellous and subperiosteal depending on the position of the lesion.

The lesion consists of a small radiolucent nidus containing nerve fibres, vascular elements and very high levels of prostaglandin which causes chronic reactive change in the surrounding bone resulting in marked surrounding periosteal sclerosis and synovitis. The excess sclerotic bone helps to point the location of the lesion during surgery. The prostaglandin is responsible for the constant, severe pain which is the most common presenting symptom.[18]

Pain is severe, unrelenting and sharp which is worse at night. It is usually nocturnal in nature and alleviated by salicylates like aspirin. Localized swelling of the soft tissue over the involved area of the bone may occur and may be tender.

Radiographic features:

Radiographically, the osteoid osteoma appears as a small, ovoid, well-circumscribed radiolucent defect, usually less than 1cm in diameter with a surrounding zone of reactive sclerosis of varying thickness. A small radiopaque central nidus may be present exhibiting some calcification. The overlying cortex becomes thickened by subperiosteal new bone formation. This all results in a target-like appearance radiographically.[22]

Histopathologic features:

The histological appearance of osteoid osteoma is characteristic. It consists of a central nidus which is composed of compact osteoid tissue, varying in degree of calcification, interspersed by a vascular connective tissue. There is definite trabeculae formation which occurs mainly in older lesions. These trabeculae are lined by osteoblasts. New bone formation occurs in the overlying periosteum. Osteoclasts and foci of bone resorption may be seen. Interstitial tissue collections of lymphocytes may also be present.[9]

Ultrastructurally, morphology of osteoblasts is similar to that of normal osteoblasts except for the mitochondria which is atypical. The morphology of osteoid osteoma is almost similar to that of osteoblastoma including atypical mitochondria. The difference between them is that in osteoid osteoma, neutral staining techniques reveal many axons through out the nidus which probably accounts for pain. Levels of prostaglandin E2 are markedly elevated in the nidus which causes vasodilatation and results in further aggravation of pain.[22]

Treatment and Prognosis:

Most cases of osteoid osteoma are treated by local excision of the lesion or curettage. The prognosis is good but a few lesions regress after incomplete excision.

CHAPTER 28

BENIGN OSTEOBLASTOMA

(Giant osteoid osteoma)

Benign osteoblastoma is a benign, vascular and progressively expansile tumor of the bone. It is an uncommon lesion that accounts for 1% of all bone tumors and about 3% of all benign bone tumors.[102]

The osteoblastic nature of the tumor often results in zones similar to those of an osteoid osteoma producing a histological resemblance. Benign osteoblastoma differs, however, in that it does not share the markedly limited growth potential of the average osteoid osteoma. Furthermore, the benign osteoblastoma frequently lacks the characteristic pain and the halo of sclerotic bone associated with osteoid osteoma. The size of the osteoblastoma is also more than 1.5 cms in its greatest dimension.

The benign osteoblastoma was first described under the name 'giant osteoid osteoma' by Dahlin and Johnson in 1954 and under the presently more accepted name by Jaffe and by Lichtenstein in 1956.[9]

Clinical Features:

Benign osteoblastoma occurs most frequently in young persons, approximately 90% under 30 years of age. However, it does occur even in elderly adults. It occurs more frequently in males with male: female ratio of 2-3:1. The lesion is characterized by pain and swelling at the tumor site.

The most common site of occurrence is the vertebral column. The first case in the jaws was reported by Borello and Sedano in 1967. It occurs in both the maxilla and mandible with almost same frequency.[103]

A small group of osteoblastomas *(aggressive osteoblastomas)* is characterized by more atypical histopathologic features and locally aggressive behavior. These tumors usually occur in older patients with most being over 30 years of age.[9]

Histological Features:

Histologically, it consists of a highly vascularized, fibro-cellular stroma in which there are abundant newly formed trabeculae of immature bone and osteoid. The mineralized material demonstrates prominent reversal lines. Proliferating osteoblasts are found lining the trabeculae of immature bone and osteoid. At the periphery of the large masses and surrounding the trabeculae, are scattered multinucleated osteoclast-like cells. These osteoblasts and osteoclasts have ample cytoplasm and hyperchromatic nuclei. The supporting stroma consists of loose fibrous connective tissue that contains scattered dilated vascular channels. Focal areas of hemorrhage are common.[102]

Microscopically, aggressive osteoblastomas are characterized by the presence of large epithelioid osteoblasts with increased mitotic activity and non trabecular sheets or lace like areas of osteoid production. On occasion, osteoblastomas may demonstrate a rich cellularity that leads to erroneous diagnosis of osteosarcoma.[22]

Malignant transformation (osteosarcoma) within a benign osteoblastoma is very rare. A *malignant osteoblastoma* has been described by Schajowicz and Lemos on the basis of a histologically i.e. more bizarre pattern of cells more abundant and often plump hyperchromatic nuclei, greater nuclear atypia and numerous giant cells. It has a better prognosis than a conventional osteosarcoma.[18]

Treatment and Prognosis:

Most cases of osteoblastoma are treated by local excision or curettage. The prognosis is good, and some lesions will regress even after incomplete excision.

CHAPTER 29

GIANT CELL TUMOR OF BONE

Giant cell tumor (GCT) of bone is also known as *osteoclastoma.* They are fairly common tumors, accounting for about 20% of all benign tumors of the bone. Most cases arise in the epiphyses of long bones, particularly the distal femur, proximal tibia, proximal humerus and distal radius. Giant cell tumors are true neoplasms that exhibit a wide spectrum of biologic behaviour from benign to malignant. The relationship between this lesion and central giant cell granuloma is controversial. Most regard the giant cell tumor as a distinct entity from central giant cell granuloma, acknowledging the very rare occurrence of giant cell tumors within the jaws.[7]

Giant cell tumor is a primary benign tumor but may evolve into a malignant tumor, usually after irradiation.

Pathogenesis:

Giant cell tumor of bone is a distinctive neoplasm of undifferentiated cells. Multinucleated giant cells apparently result from fusion of the proliferating mononuclear cells, and although they are a constant and prominent part of this tumor, the giant cells are probably of less significance than the mononuclear cells. The exact cell of origin of this neoplasm is still unknown. Several immunohistochemical studies have suggested that the mononuclear cells are of histiocytic origin and that the giant cells arise from their fusion.[18]

Clinical features:

They occur most often between the ages of 20 and 40 years, with a slight female predominance. Giant cell tumors, although rare, have been reported in the jaws. Other sites of involvement in the head and neck include the sphenoid, ethmoid, and temporal bones. Giant cell tumors are most often seen in the third and fourth decades of life.[7]

This lesion may exhibit a wide range of biologic behaviour and thus may present a variety of clinical features. Benign variants may exhibit slow growth and bone expansion. Rapid malignant variety or large tumors may produce rapid growth. Pain of variable severity is almost always a predominant symptom. Less common symptoms are weakness, limitation of motion of the joint and pathological fracture.[104]

Malignant giant cell tumor:

Giant cell tumor is known to evolve into malignant tumor. McGrath (1972) classified such tumors into three types: primary, evolutionary and secondary. "Primary" is for tumors that are malignant from outset, "evolutionary" for typical tumors that progress to a malignant form within a short period and "secondary" for typical tumors that undergo sarcomatous changes after a relatively long symptom-free period, and usually develop after irradiation (post irradiation malignancy).[105]

Histological features:

On gross inspection the lesion is well circumscribed and often has a granular hemorrhagic appearance. The expanded portion is partially or completely encased in a thin shell of bone. The neoplastic tissue is firm and friable. It is often grayish, with either a pinkish or a brownish tint. Focal areas of cystic degeneration, of yellow-brown color, and hemorrhagic areas that are red or dark brown, depending on the age of the haemorrhage, are usually present.

The microscopic hallmark of this neoplasm is the presence of a large number of multinucleated giant cells that are regularly scattered throughout the tumor mass. The giant cells of this neoplasm have an abundant acidophilic cytoplasm and as many as 100 nuclei. Their light microscopic, enzymatic, histochemical, and fine structural features are similar to those of normal osteoclasts. Thus acid phosphatase activity is very high and a large number of mitochondria are present in the cytoplasm. Because of these similarities, giant cell tumor of bone is also known as osteoclastoma.

The second microscopic component of the giant cell tumor is *stromal cell.* Although far less spectacular than the giant cell when examined under the microscope, it is probably the basic tumor element. It is certainly more important numerically than the giant cell. The relative number and appearance of these stromal cells correlates with the clinical evolution. In locally aggressive and metastasizing lesions, one often gets the impression that the stromal cell component has taken over the neoplasm.

The stromal cells of a typical giant cell tumor are medium sized and oval or spindle shaped, with rather plump nuclei and ill-defined acidophilic cytoplasm. Mononuclear macrophages are also present in large numbers, but they probably are nonneoplastic and an expression of the host reaction to the tumor. The stroma is richly vascularized and contains a small amount of collagen. In about a third of the cases, foci of osteoid or bone formation of reactive appearance are found. Under the electron microscope the stromal cells are seen to contain a well-developed granular endoplasmic reticulum. Their appearance is reminiscent of a fibroblast or an osteoblast.

Treatment & prognosis:

Surgical excision is the treatment of choice for giant cell tumors. Giant cell tumors are aggressive lesions. As much as 60% recur after curettage, and about 10% result in distant metastasis, usually to the lungs.[2]

CHAPTER 30

HODGKIN'S DISEASE

Thomas Hodgkin first described Hodgkin's disease in 1832. It is a potentially curable malignant lymphoma with distinct histology, biologic behavior, and clinical characteristics.[18] The etiology of HD is unknown. Infectious agents, especially the Epstein-Barr virus (EBV), may be involved in the pathogenesis. Patients with HIV infection have a higher incidence of HD compared to the population without HIV infection. Genetic predisposition may play a role in the pathogenesis.[18]

Clinical Features:

Age-specific incidence rates have a bimodal distribution in both genders, peaking in young adults (aged 15-34 years) and older individuals (>55 years). HD is more common in males than in females, particularly evident in children.

The first manifestation in the majority of cases is painless enlargement of one or more cervical lymph nodes. Palpable painless lymphadenopathy occurs in the cervical area (60-80%), axilla (6-20%), and less commonly, in the inguinal area (6-20%) and Waldeyer ring or occipital nodes. The nodes are usually firm and rubbery in consistency and the overlying skin is normal. Constitutional symptoms such as unexplained weight loss, fever, night sweats are present in about 40% of patients. Chest pain, cough, and/or shortness of breath may be present due to a large mediastinal mass or lung involvement. Alcohol induced pain at sites of nodal disease is specific for HD.[18]

Oral Manifestations:

Hodgkin's disease is primarily a disease of lymph nodes and the oral cavity could be involved secondarily. A case of Hodgkin's disease secondarily involving the mandible and overlying alveolar mucosa has been reported by Forman and Wesson.[18]

Histologic Features:

1. Nodular sclerosis Hodgkin's disease comprises 60-80% of all cases. The morphology shows a nodular pattern. The broad bands of fibrosis divide the node into 'nodules'. The capsule is thickened. The characteristic cell is the lacunar-type RS cell, which has a monolobated or multi lobated nucleus and a small nucleolus with abundant and pale cytoplasm. It is commonly observed in adolescents and young adults, usually involves the mediastinum and supradiaphragmatic sites.
2. Mixed-cellularity Hodgkin's disease comprises 15-30%. Histologically, the infiltrate is usually diffuse. RS cells are of the classic type (large, with bilobate, double or multiple nuclei, and a large eosinophilic inclusion like nucleolus). It commonly affects the abdominal lymph nodes and spleen.
3. Lymphocyte-depleted Hodgkin's disease makes up less than 1%. The infiltrate in lymphocyte-depleted Hodgkin disease (LDHD) is diffuse and often appears hypocellular. Large numbers of RS cells and bizarre sarcomatous variants are present. It is associated with older age and HIV positivity. Patients usually present with advanced-stage disease.
4. Lymphocyte-rich classic Hodgkin's disease comprises 5%. In this type of HD, RS cells of the classic or lacunar type are observed, with a background infiltrate of lymphocytes. Clinically, the presentation and survival patterns are similar to those for mixed-cellularity Hodgkin disease.
5. Nodular lymphocyte-predominant Hodgkin's disease constitutes 5%. A variant of RS cells, the lymphocytic and histiocytic cells (L&H), or popcorn cells (their nuclei resemble an exploded kernel of corn), are seen within a background of inflammatory cells, predominantly benign lymphocytes.[18]

Treatment and Prognosis:

Radiation therapy and combination chemotherapy have been clearly shown to be effective in the management of Hodgkin's disease. The most important prognostic determinants are the histologic type and the clinical stage of the disease. The lymphocyte predominant type has the most favorable prognosis, followed by nodular sclerosis, mixed cellularity and lymphocyte depletion, the least favorable. Localized (Stage I) disease has a much better prognosis than disseminated (Stage IV) disease.[18]

CHAPTER 31

CENTRAL HEMANGIOMA

Central hemangioma of bone are vascular malformations that, when seen in the jaws, can mimic both odontogenic and nonodontogenic lesions. On surgical intervention the hemorrhage is difficult to control.

Clinical Features:

More than half of the central hemangiomas of the jaws occur in the mandible, especially the posterior region. The lesion occurs approximately twice as often in females as in males. The peak age of discovery is the second decade of life.

A firm, slow-growing, asymmetric expansion of the mandible or maxilla is the most common patient complaint. Spontaneous gingival bleeding around teeth in the area of the hemangioma may also be noted. Paresthesia or pain, vertical mobility of involved teeth, bruits or pulsation of large lesions may be detected. Trophic effects of the hemangioma on adjacent hard and soft tissues are also common. Radiographically, more than half of jaw hemangiomas occur as multilocular radiolucencies that have a characteristic soap bubble appearance.[9]

Histopathological features:

Hemangiomas of bone represent a proliferation of blood vessels. Most intrabony hemangiomas are of the cavernous type (large-caliber vessels). Fewer are of the capillary type (small-caliber vessels). Bone is involved resulting in reactive osteoclastic and osteoblastic remodeling. The cortical and trabecular bone is thin and numerous osteoclasts are identified at interface between vascular tissue and bone.[18]

Treatment and Prognosis:

Methods used in the treatment of hemangioma of bone include surgery, radiation therapy, sclerosing agents, cryotherapy, and presurgical embolization techniques

CHAPTER 32

MISCELLANEOUS LESIONS

MASSIVE OSTEOLYSIS

Massive osteolysis or GORHAM's disease was first defined as a specific entity by Gorham in 1955. It develops in any part of the skeleton but the process affecting the facial bones was first presented by Romer in 1924. The mandible is one of the most common bones concerned and its invasion undergoes partial or complete dissolution and spreads across joints to contiguous bones or involves the adjacent soft tissues.[106]

Clinical features:

There are two phases in the massive osteolysis. The first is the active form of bone resorption and its progression. Clinically, it produces often the loss of the teeth, pathological fractures with mild pain; less frequently tissue swelling and sepsis. The recurrent infections may reach the adjacent organs such as the middle ear, inner ear and meanings. The second phase represents the latent form. Moreover, bone defects are associated with both several and grave dysfunctions consisting of mastication, swallowing, speaking and respiratory functions and a notable facial deformity. The course and duration of the phases cannot be foreseen and the active form can last for months or years.[106]

Histopathological features:

The histopathological characteristic of the GORHAM's disease is the replacement of bone tissue by intrafibrous connective tissue containing many thin-walled vessels or anastomosing vascular spaces, including lymphatic capillaries; termed histologically hemangiomatosis as used by Stout. Osteoclasts are generally but not always present and their number is, however, usually low. [106]

Treatment:

Surgical intervention and radiotherapy are the suggested methods of treatment.

CHAPTER 33

SPITZ NEVUS

The spitzs nevus (SN) is named after Sophie Spitz, who first described it in 1948. It is also called benign juvenile melanoma or spindle epithelioid cell nevus. It is a benign tumour found predominantly in children and adolescents. The condition is clinically significant in view of the difficulties in differentiating it from malignant melanoma (MM). Its incidence is less than 1% of all nevi in children. Majority of SN are spindle cell type but epithelioid cell type is uncommon.[107]

Clinical features:

Clinically the nevus is usually asymptomatic, solitary, dome- shaped, smooth - surfaced, pink or tan, sometimes brown or even black lesion. Majority of Spitz nevi are situated on the head and legs (56.5%); the number on the trunk and arms is smaller (38%). In terms of their architectural pattern SN is usually symmetrical, less than 1 cm in diameter.

Histological features:

Epidermal hyperplasia is prominent in SN. Usually there is little or no pagetoid spread of lesional cells into epidermis in SN. There is blunt pushing margin. Single attenuated cells or files of single cells are dispersed between reticular dermal collagen bundles which are highly characteristic of SN.

Bizarre giant cells may be present, which have regular nuclei of similar size. Lack of atypical mitosis and no mitosis and no mitotic activity favours the diagnosis of SN. Melanin is generally completely or nearly absent in SN (70%).[107]

Treatment:

Because of the difficulty of making an absolutely certain differentiation between SN and MM, it is advisable as a precautionary measure that all lesions diagnosed as SN be excised in persons at or beyond puberty, particularly because such lesions are usually small. [107]

CHAPTER 34

XANTHOMAS

Xanthomas are tumor-like collections of foamy histiocytes within the dermis. They may be associated with familial or acquired disorders resulting in hyperlipidemia, with lymphoproliferative malignancies, or without any underlying disorder.[8]

Clinical features:

The age of occurrence widely varies from 2-89 years. But most oral cases occur in middle-aged persons with mean age of 40-50 years. No gender predilection is apparent. The lesion may occur at any site but most preferred site is the alveolar ridge or gingiva, followed by the buccal mucosa, palate, floor of mouth, lip and lower mucobuccal fold.

This occurs as a solitary lesion, normal or reddish in colour, with rough pebbly surface. It may be sessile or pedunculated, 2mm-1.5cm in size and is asymptomatic.[18]

Histological features:

Variable degree of parakeratosis with hyperparakeratosis present in the crypts between papillae. The rete ridges are extremely elongated and uniform. The most characteristic feature is the presence of large foam cells in the connective tissue papillae between the epithelial pegs. These are the fat laden macrophages. A slight inflammatory infiltrate may be present beneath the lesion.[18]

Treatment:

Local surgical excision is almost always curative. Recurrence is rare

UNIT 3
CONCLUSION

Giant cell lesion of the maxillofacial skeleton and other bones are a controversial matter and uncertainity still exists regarding their basic pathology and biologic behaviour.

Fifty years ago, giant cell lesions of the jaws were generally diagnosed as giant cell tumors and these lesions were widely considered to be similar to those that occurred in the extragnathic skeleton.

Considering the very diverse clinical behavior, it is possible that some lesions are merely reactive in origin while in others an as yet undiscovered genetic abnormality might play a role.Further research is needed to elucidate this question.

Despite the difficulty in predicting the behaviour of giant cell lesions of jaws, a consideration of clinical, radiographic and histopathological features helps to determine the appropriate therapy. Therefore, the important reason for studying the pathobiology of lesions is to provide a rational basis for the application of novel therapeutic agents.

REFERENCES

1. Wakefield, Denis, Kumar R, Kotla. Inflammation: Chronic. 10.1038/npg.els.0000944.
2. Kissane JM, Anderson WAD. Anderson's Pathology. 8th edition, C.V. Mosby Company (2004).
3. Postlethwaite AE, Jackson BK, Beachey EH, Kang AH. Formation of multinucleated giant cells from human monocyte precursors. J of Exp Med (1982); 155: 168-178.
4. Chambers TJ. Multinucleate Giant Cells. J of Pathol (1978); 126: 125-148.
5. Liu B, Yu S-F, Li T-J. Multinucleated giant cells in various forms of giant cell containing lesions of the jaws express features of osteoclasts. J Oral Pathol Med (2003); 32: 367–375.
6. Mariano M, Spector WG. The formation and properties of macrophage polykaryons (inflammatory giant cells). J of Pathol (1973); 113(1): 1-19.
7. Anderson JM. Multinucleated giant cells. Current Opinion in Hematology (2000); 7: 40-47.
8. Kumar V, Cotran RS, Robbins SL. Basic Pathology. 7th edition, Elsevier New Delhi (2003).
9. Neville BW, Damm DD, Allen CM, Bouquot JE. Oral and Maxillofacial Pathology. 2nd edition, Elsevier New Delhi (2002).
10. Philipsen HP, Reichart PA. Odontogenic Tumors and Allied Lesions. Quintessence Publishing Company Ltd. (2003).
11. El-Labban NG. Intravascular fibrin thrombi and endothelial cell damage in central giant cell granuloma. J Oral Pathol Med (1997); 26: 1-5.
12. Abrams B, Shear M. A histological comparison of the giant cells in the central giant cell granuloma of the jaws and the giant cell tumor of long bone. J of Oral Path (1974); 3: 217-223.
13. Speight PM. Giant cell lesions of the jaws: Guest Editorial. Oral Diseases (1995); 1: 6-7.

14. Chattopadhyay A. Giant Cells and Giant Cell Lesions of the oral cavity. JIDA (1995); 66(11):326-327.

15. Antonio Nanci. Tencate's Oral Histology: Development, Structure and Function. 6th edition, Elsevier New Delhi (2006).

16. Harokopakis-Hajishengallis E. Physiologic root resorption in primary teeth: molecular and histological events. J of Oral Science (2007); 49(1): 1-12.

17. Trope M. Luxation injuries and external root resorption -- etiology, treatment, and prognosis. J of the California Dental Ass (2000); 28(11): 860-866.

18. Shafer, Hine, Levy. Text book of Oral Pathology. 5th edition, Elsevier New Delhi (2006).

19. Niikuni N, Seki N, Sato K, Nasu D, Shirakawa T. Traumatic injury to permanent tooth resulting in complete root resorption: a case report.

J of Oral Science (2007); 49(4): 341-344.

20. Pizzo G, Licata ME, Guiglia R, Giuliana G. Root resorption and orthodontic treatment. Minerva Stomatol (2007); 56: 31-44.

21. Gunraj M. Dental root resorption.Oral Surg Oral Med Oral Pathol Oral Radiol Endod (1999); 88: 647-653.

22. Regezi JA, Sciubba JJ, Jordan RCK. Oral Pathology Clinical Pathologic Correlations. 4th edition, Elsevier New Delhi (2003).

23. Bork K, Hoede N, Korting GW, Burgdorf WHC, Young SK. Disease of the Oral Mucosa and the Lips. 2nd edition, W.B. Saunders Company (1996).

24. Soares AB, Gonzaga HFS, Jorge MA, Barraviera SRCS. Oral Manifestations of Syphilis: A Review. J Venom Anim Toxins incl Trop Dis (2004); 10(1): 2-9.

25. Goh B. Syphilis. Medicine (2005), 33(10): 48-51.

26. Leao JC, Gueiros LA, Porter SR. Oral manifestations of syphilis. Clinics (2006); 61(2):161-166.

27. Lautenschlager S. Cutaneous manifestations of Syphilis: recognition and management. Am J Clin Dermatol (2006); 7 (5): 291-304.

28. Lichtenstein L, Jaffe HL. Fibrous Dysplasia of Bone. Arch Surg (1938); 36: 777-816.

29. de Abre MAMM, Michalany NS, Weckx LLM, Pimentel DRN, Hirata CHW, de Avelar Alchorne MM. The oral mucosa in leprosy: a clinical and histopathological study. Rev Bras Otorrinolaringol (2006); 72(3): 312-316.

30. Motta ACF, Komesu MC, Silva CHL, Arruda D, Simao JCL, Zenha EMR, Furini RB, Foss NT. Leprosy-specific oral lesions: A report of three cases. Med Oral Patol Oral Cir Bucal (2008);13(8): 479-482.

31. Fucci da Costa AP, Augusto da Costa Nery J, Wan-del-Rey de Oliveira ML, Cuzzi T, Ramos-e-Silva M. Oral lesions in leprosy. Indian J Dermatol Venereol Leprol (2003); 69: 381-385.

32. Arduino PG, Porter SR. Herpes Simplex Virus Type I infection: overview on relevant clinico-pathological features. J Oral Pathol Med (2008); 37: 107-121.

33. Ananthnarayan R. Textbook of Microbiology. 5th edition, Orient longman Ltd. (1996).

34. Tateishi K, Toh Y, Minagawa H, Tashiro H. Detection of Herpes simplex virus (HSV) in the saliva from 1,000 oral surgery outpatients by the polymerase chain reaction (PCR) and virus isolation. J Oral Pathol Med (1994); 23: 80-84.

35. Scott DA, Coulter WA, Biagioni PA, O'Neill H, Lamey P-J. Detection of herpes simplex virus type 1 shedding in the oral cavity by polymerase chain reaction and enzyme-linked immunosorbent assay at the prodromal stage of recrudescent herpes labialis. J Oral Pathol Med (1997); 26: 305-309.

36. Siegel MA. Diagnosis and management of recurrent herpes simplex infections. J Am Dent Assoc (2002); 133: 1245-1249.

37. Gilbert SC. Oral shedding of herpes virus type I in immunocompetent persons. J Oral Pathol Med (2006); 35: 548-553.

38. Hedner E, Vahlne A, Bergstrom T, Hirsch JM. Recrudescence of herpes simplex virus type 1 in latently infected rats after trauma to oral tissues. J Oral Pathol Med (1993); 22: 214-220.

39. Arduino PG, Porter SR. Oral and perioral herpes simplex virus type I (HSV-I) infection: review of its management. Oral Diseases (2006); 12: 254-270.

40. Opstelten W, van Loon AM, Schuller M, van Wijck AJM, van Essen GA, Moons KGM, Verheij TJM. Clinical Diagnosis of Herpes Zoster in Family Practice. Ann Fam Med (2007); 5: 305-309.

41. Gupta LK, Singhi MK. Tzanck smear: A useful diagnostic tool. Indian J Dermatol Venereol Leprol (2005); 71: 295-299.

42. Lambert EM, Strasswimmer J, Lazova R, Antaya RJ. Cytomegalovirus ulcer: successful treatment with valganciclovir. Arch Dermatol (2004); 140: 1199-1120.

43. Mattes FM, McLaughlin JE, Emery VC, Clark DA, Griffiths PD. Histopathological detection of owl's eye inclusions is still specific for cytomegalovirus in the era of human herpesviruses 6 and 7. J Clin Pathol (2000); 53: 612-614.

44. Gilbert SC. Oral shedding of herpes virus type I in immunocompetent persons.

J Oral Pathol Med (2006); 35: 548-553.

45. Maxillary necrosis by mucormycosis. A case report and literature review. Med Oral Patol Oral Cir Bucal (2007); 12: E360-364.

46. Frater JL, Hall GS, Procop GW. Histologic Features of Zygomycosis: Emphasis on Perineural Invasion and Fungal Morphology. Arch Pathol Lab Med (2001); 125: 375-378.

47. Denning DW. Invasive Aspergillosis. Clinical Infectious Diseases (1998); 26: 781-805.

48. Dubey A, Patwardhan RV, Sampth S, Santosh V, Kolluri S, Nanda A. Intracranial fungal granuloma: analysis of 40 patients and review of the literature. Surgical Neurology (2005); 63: 254-260.

49. Ray R, Singh ZN, Wasir HS, Chopra P. Isolated Cardiac Aspergillosis. Indian Heart J (2001); 53: 505-507.

50. Milian MA, Bagan JV, Jimenez Y, Perez A, Scully C. Oral leishmaniasis in a HIV-positive patient. Report of a case involving the palate. Oral Diseases (2002), 8: 59-61.

51. Chaudhry Z, Barrett AW, Corbett E, French PD, Zakrzewska JM. Oral mucosal leishmaniasis as a presenting feature of HIV infection and its management. J Oral Pathol Med (1999); 28: 43-46.

52. Motta ACF, Lopes MA, Ito FA, Carlos-Bregni R, de Almeida OP, Roselino AM. Oral leishmaniasis: a clinicopathological study of 11 cases. Oral Diseases (2007); 13: 335-340.

53. Mabey D, Peeling RW. Lymphogranuloma venereum. Sex Transm Infect (2002); 78: 90–92.

54. Mehta V, Balachandran C, Bhat S, Geetha V, Fernanades D. Nasal NK/T cell lymphoma presenting as a midline lethal granuloma. Indian J Dermatol Venereol Leprol (2008); 74: 145-147.

55. Borges A, James Fink J, Villablanca P, Eversole R, Lufkin R. Destructive Lesions of the Sinonasal Tract: Simplified Terminology Based on Histopathologic Criteria. Am J Neuroradiol (2000); 21:331-336.

56. Lilly J, Juhlin T, Lew D, Vincent S, Lilly G. Wegener's granulomatosis presenting as oral lesions: A case report. Oral Surg Oral Med Oral Pathol Oral Radiol Endod (1998); 85: 153-157.

57. Akikusa JD, Schneider R, Harvey EA, Hebert D, Thorner PS, Laxer RM, Silverman ED. Clinical Features and Outcome of Pediatric Wegener's Granulomatosis. Arthritis Rheum (2007); 57(5): 837-844.

58. Abu-Hilal M, Abu-Hilal M, McPhail MJW, Zeidan B, Bryant T, Bateman A, Johnson CD. Acute Pancreatitis as the First Presentation of Wegener's Granulomatosis. J Pancreas (2008); 9(3): 300-304.

59. Yao X, Alvarado Y, Brackeen J, Jumper C, Cobos E. Plasma Cell Granuloma: A case report of multiple lesions in the lung and review of the literature. Am J Med Sci (2007); 334(5): 402-406.

60. Buccoliero AM, Caldarella A, Santucci M, Ammannati F, Mennonna P, Taddei A, Taddei GL. Plasma Cell Granuloma—An Enigmatic Lesion. Arch Pathol Lab Med (2003); 127: 220-223.

61. Suresh L, Radfar L. Oral sarcoidosis: a review of literature. Oral Diseases (2005); 11: 138-145.

62. Judson MA. Sarcoidosis: clinical presentation, diagnosis, and approach to treatment. Am J Med Sci (2008); 335(1): 26-33.

63. Pierce TB, Margolis M, Razzuk MA. Sarcoidosis: still a mystery? BUMC Proceedings (2001); 14: 8-12.

64. Camacho-Alonso F, Bermejo-Fenoll A, Lopez-Jornet P. Miescher's cheilitis granulomatosa. A presentation of five cases. Med Oral Patol Oral Cir Bucal (2004); 9: 425-429.

65. Sapp JP, Eversole LR, Wysocki GP. Contemporary Oral and Maxillofacial Pathology. 2nd edition, Mosby Company (2004).

66. Goncalves DU, deCastro MM, Galvao CP, Brandao AZ, deCastro MC, Lambertucci JR. Cheilitis granulomatosa associated with melkersson-rosenthal syndrome. Rev Bras Otorrinolaringol (2007); 73(1): 138-139.

67. Gungormus M, Akgul HM. Central giant cell granuloma of the jaws: A clinical and radiologic study. J Contemp Dent Pract (2003); (4)3: 87-97.

68. Mabey D, Peeling RW. Lymphogranuloma venereum. Sex Transm Infect (2002); 78: 90–92.

69. Vered M, Buchner A, Dayan D. Giant cell granuloma of the jawbones – a proliferative vascular lesion? Immunohistochemical study with vascular endothelial growth factor and basic fibroblast growth factor. J Oral Pathol Med (2006); 35: 613-619.

70. Stavropoulos F, Katz J. Central giant cell granulomas: A systematic review of the radiographic characteristics with the addition of 20 new cases. Dentomaxillofacial Radiology (2002); 31: 213-217.

71. Farrier SL, Farrier JN, Smart MK, Nash ES. A 10-year review of the occurrence and treatment of central giant cell granulomas, in a District

General Hospital. J Oral Pathol Med (2006); 35: 332-337.

72. Kaffe I, Ardekian L, Taicher S, Littner M, Buchner A. Radiologic features of central giant cell granuloma of the jaws.Oral Surg Oral Med Oral Pathol Oral Radiol Endod (1996); 8: 720-726.

73. Chaparro-Avendano AV, Berini-Aytes L, Gay Escoda C. Peripheral giant cell granuloma. A report of five cases and review of the literature. Med Oral Patol Oral Cir Bucal (2005); 10: 48-57.

74. Bastian TS, Mehta R. Peripheral giant cell granuloma. KSDJ (2005); 24: 59-63.

75. Bodner L, Peist M, Gatot A, Fliss DM. Growth potential of peripheral giant cell granuloma. Oral Surg Oral Med Oral Pathol Oral Radiol Endod (1997); 83: 548-551.

76. Gandara JM, Pacheco JL, Gandara P Blanco A, Garcia A, Madrinan P, Somoza M. Peripheral giant-cell granuloma. Review of 13 cases. Medicina Oral (2002); 7: 254-259

77. Mighell AJ, Robinson PA, Hume WJ. Peripheral giant cell granuloma: a clinical study of 77 cases from 62 patients, and literature review. Oral Diseases (1995); 1: 12- 19.

78. Pandolfi PJ, Felefli S, Flaitz CM, Johnson JV. An aggressive peripheral giant cell granuloma in a child. J Clin Pediatr Dent (1999); 23(4): 353-355.

79. Aterman K, Remmele W, Smith M. Karl Touton and His "Xanthelasmatic Giant Cell". Am J of Derma (1988); 10(3): 257-269.

80. Mooney GC, McMahon J, Ward SE, Davidson LE, North S. Management of central giant cell granuloma: discussion of two cases. International Journal of Paediatric Dentistry (2007); 17: 139-144.

81. Pandolfi PJ, Felefli S, Flaitz CM, Johnson JV. An aggressive peripheral giant cell granuloma in a child. J Clin Pediatr Dent (1999); 23(4): 353-355.

82. Carvalho YR, Loyola AM, Gomez RS, Araujo VC. Peripheral giant cell granuloma. An immunohistochemical and ultrastructural study. Oral Diseases (1995); 1: 20-25.

83. Eslami K, Anderson T. Clinical presentation of secondary hyperparathyroidism. Australian Doctor (2002); 7: 322-325.

84. Sharma P, Parikh K, Chhabra A, Kapadia B, Vohra K, Verma S. Classical Case of Primary Hyperparathyroidism. Ind J Radiol Imag (2005); 15(4): 485-487.

85. Brannon RB, Fowler CB. Benign Fibrous Lesions: A Review of Current Concepts. Advances in Anatomic Pathology (2001); 8(3): 126-143.

86. Krishnakumar R, Priyadarshini R, Elumalai K, Rangarajan GK, Ayyappan. Paget's disease and bone scan: A case report. World J Nucl Med (2006); 5: 201-204.

87. Fraser WD. Paget's disease of bone. CPD Rheumatology (2001); 2(1): 8-13.

88. Eversole LR, Rovin S. Reactive lesions of the gingiva. J Oral Path (1972); 1: 30-38.

89. Jeffrey S, Brien O, Kevin E, Mark H, Chandra M. Paget's disease of bone in an Indian patient: genetic and environmental factors. Journal of Clinical Rheumatology (2002); 8(4): 212-216.

90. Campos E, Gomez RS. Immunocytochemical Study of Giant Cell Fibroma. Braz Dent J (1999); 10(2): 89-92.

91. Culberson JD, Enterline HT. Pseudosarcomatous Fasciitis: A Distinctive Clinical-Pathologic Entity; Report of Five Cases. Annals of Surgery (1960): 235-241.

92. Tamarit-Borras M, Delgado-Molina E, Berini-Aytes L, Gay-Escoda C. Removal of hyperplastic lesions of the oral cavity: A retrospective study of 128 cases. Med Oral Patol Oral Cir Bucal (2005); 10: 151-162.

93. Pilolli GP, Lucchese A, Scivetti M, Maiorano E, Favia G. Traumatic ulcerative granuloma with stromal eosinophilia of the oral mucosa: histological and immunohistochemical analysis of three cases. Minerva Stomatol (2007); 56: 73-79.

94. Hirshberg A, Amariglio N, Akrish S, Yahalom R, Rosenbaum H, Okon E, Kaplan I. Traumatic ulcerative granuloma with stromal eosinophilia: A reactive lesion of the oral mucosa. Am J Clin Pathol (2006); 126: 522-529.

95. Shear M, Speight PM. Cysts of the Oral and Maxillofacial Regions. 4th edition, Blackwell Munksgaard (2007).

96. Prasad S, Raghaviah AM, Sharma N, Einstein A, Saraswathi TR. Aneurysmal bone cyst of the mandible: Report of a case and review of the literature. J Oral Maxillofac Pathol (2007); 11: 38-41.

97. Kransdorf MJ, Sweet DE. Aneurysmal Bone Cyst: concept, controversy, clinical presentation, and imaging. AJR (1995); 164: 573-580.

98. Mendenhall WM, Zlotecki RA, Gibbs CP, Reith JD, Scarborough MT, Mendenhall NP. Aneurysmal Bone Cyst. . Am J Clin Oncol (2006); 29: 311-315.

99. Dabska M, Buraczewski J. Aneurysmal Bone Cyst: Pathology, Clinical Course and Radiologic Appearances. Cancer (1969): 23; 371-389.

100. Eshghyar N, Jalayer-Nadery N, Ashery R. Calcifying Odontogenic Cyst: An analysis of thirty-six cases. Acta Medica Iranica (2006); 44(1): 59-62.

101. Rajkumar K, Kamal K, Sathish MR, Leena S. Calcifying odontogenic cyst. J Oral Maxillofac Pathol (2004); 8: 99-103.

102. Durmaz R, Bozoglu H, Kabukcuoglu S, Vardareli E. Osteoblastoma of the Cervical Spine. Histopathological and Radiological Correlation. Turkish Neurosurgery (1996); 6: 88-92.

103. Chun KA, Cho IH, Won KJ, Lee HW, Choi JH, Ahn JC, Shin DS. Osteoblastoma as a cause of osteomalacia assessed by bone scan. Annals of Nuclear Medicine (2003); 17(5): 411-414.

104. Eckardt JJ, Grogan TJ. Giant Cell Tumor of Bone. Clinical Orthopedics and Related Research (1986); 204: 45-58.

105. Hashimoto K, Hatori M, Hosaka M, Watanabe M, Hasegawa T, Kokubun S. Osteosarcoma arising from giant cell tumor of bone ten years after primary surgery: A case report and review of the literature.

Tohoku J Exp Med (2006); 208: 157-162.

106. Benhalima H, Lazrak A, Boulaich M, Mezahi M, Ourlai A, Kzadri M, Amarti A, Saidi M. Massive osteolysis of the maxillo-facial bones: case report and review of the literature. Odonto-Stomatologie Tropicale (2001); 96: 35-40.

107. Mohan H, Chopra R, Bhardwaj K, Bhard. Spitz nevus. Indian J Dermatol Venereol Leprol (1998); 64: 240-242.

www.ingramcontent.com/pod-product-compliance
Ingram Content Group UK Ltd.
Pitfield, Milton Keynes, MK11 3LW, UK
UKHW061539190726
13845UKWH00031B/1113

9 788198 495860